BETWEEN SICKNESS AND HEALTH

Between Sickness and Health is about illness rather than disease, and recovery rather than cure. The book argues that illness is an experience, represented by the feeling that 'I am not myself'. From the book's phenomenological point of view, feelings of illness cannot be 'unreal' or 'fake', whatever their biological basis, nor need they be categorised as 'physical', 'psychosomatic' or 'psychiatric'.

The book challenges the disease-centred ethos of medicine and medical education. It demonstrates that a clearer conception of illness, as distinct from disease, is therapeutic. The feeling that 'I am once again myself' can return, in some degree, whatever state the body is in. Resilience becomes more available when it is seen as a set of personal skills that can be developed, rather than as an inborn trait. Possibilities of wellness are enhanced by recognising that medical and other therapies can either support or impede recovery, as can human relationships and the socio-political environment.

The book's many clinical examples are drawn from the author's broad experience as a neurologist, rehabilitation physician and systemic family therapist. *Between Sickness and Health* will be useful for students, practitioners and academics, and also for anyone who has been or might one day be ill.

Christopher D. Ward is Emeritus Professor of Rehabilitation Medicine at the University of Nottingham, UK. He is also a UKCP-accredited systemic psychotherapist. He edited *Meanings of ME: Interpersonal and Social Dimensions of Chronic Fatigue*, 2015.

BETWEEN SICKNESS AND HEALTH

The Landscape of Illness and Wellness

Christopher D. Ward

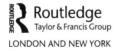

LONDON AND NEW YORK

First published 2020
by Routledge
2 Park Square, Milton Park, Abingdon, Oxon OX14 4RN

and by Routledge
52 Vanderbilt Avenue, New York, NY 10017

Routledge is an imprint of the Taylor & Francis Group, an informa business

© 2020 Christopher D. Ward

British Library Cataloguing in Publication Data
A catalogue record for this book is available from the British Library

Library of Congress Cataloging-in-Publication Data
A catalog record has been requested for this book

ISBN: 978-1-138-59286-5 (hbk)
ISBN: 978-1-138-59287-2 (pbk)
ISBN: 978-0-429-48975-4 (ebk)

Typeset in Bembo
by Taylor & Francis Books

CONTENTS

ILLUSTRATIONS

Figures

Tables

ACKNOWLEDGEMENTS

Thanks to the patients and their families for what they have taught me; to many colleagues, particularly Lindsay Maclellan, Alison Smith and Margaret Phillips for what I have picked up through working with them clinically; to Lawrence Weaver, for inspiring and informative ruminations about medicine and history; to my brother Jon Ward, for making me more mindful of non-western perspectives; to Evan Sedgwick-Jell for political perspectives; to Grace McInnes and her team at Routledge for encouragement and advice; and to my wife Harriet for both tolerating and inspiring this project.

PREFACE

This book re-examines the idea of illness. Its point of departure is a suffering individual – a particular person in a particular predicament. But what can I, writing primarily from the perspective of a former physician, say about illness that ill people cannot say for themselves? Doctors translate illness into 'a symbolic system, . . . facilitating as well as constraining understanding and action'.[1] Put less starkly, doctors 'can call to our body, can tell us if its anger is serious or will soon be appeased'.[2] A doctor does this without necessarily entering those deeper recesses of illness experience where everybody's language fails. Anatole Broyard gives me heart, however, in his description of the kind of doctor he ideally wanted when he was diagnosed with prostatic cancer. He wrote that the doctor turns the raw materials of illness into 'a poem of diagnosis'. I believe that a patient and a doctor, and usually a family as well, are joint witnesses to illness. Doctors gain something of an inside view of the tragedy and ugliness of illness, and occasionally other less sinister things. Broyard hoped his doctor would enjoy him – with a little irony perhaps, but not with scare quotes. It is an odd truth that the tension a clinician feels at the end of a working day is often mixed with a sense of reassurance that I think comes from the goodness that can emerge from almost the worst of situations. Broyard hoped his doctor would 'read' him as literature.[3] In this book I have been offering my readings of peoples' experiences of illness.

I read with the eyes firstly of a physician, secondly of a family therapist, and thirdly of someone with a few relevant personal experiences of illness. At the same time, I have the critical eye of an academic. I admit to a desire 'not to be a slave of one science, or dwell altogether in one subject, as most do, but to rove abroad', which I fear has made me 'a ranging spaniel, that barks at every bird he sees, leaving his game. . . .'.[4] What I have wanted to do, in as scholarly a way as possible, is to point out the many different birds that are up there, in the landscape of illness and recovery.

When I say scholarly, I mean close reading and critical thinking. However, I have not comprehensively described any single aspect of this vast subject. My aim has been to indicate a range of relevant lines of thought. Wikipedia has certainly been my friend at times. If I, too, have 'confusedly tumbled over divers authors in our libraries', I hope to have made some suggestive connections between the many perspectives from which illness can be contemplated. Descartes' advice at the beginning of one of his essays could be adapted. He asked readers to 'take the trouble, before reading this, to have cut open in front of them the heart of some large animal which has lungs'.[5] As you read this book, a less messy option would be to have access to more definitive sources of medical sociology, medical anthropology, medical history, health psychology and other academic domains that are relevant to illness.

Notes

1 Bury 1982
2 Proust 1920/1982 p. 308
3 *The Patient Examines the Doctor* 1992; Broyard died in 1989, the year after his diagnosis
4 Robert Burton *The Anatomy of Melancholy*, 1621
5 Descartes 1637/1968 p. 66

A NOTE TO PATIENTS, CLIENTS AND FAMILIES

I owe most of what I know about illness to what you have told me. There are too many of you, stretching over too long a period of time, for it to be possible for me to ask your permission to translate my observations and experiences into a book. I have had to think hard about how to represent your lives here, because I am anxious not to break the trust you placed in me.

I will be writing about my perceptions of your experience , and I will be reporting what you said to me. However, no-one will recognise you, and you would be very unlikely to recognise yourself, because in the stories I tell I have gone to great lengths to alter things about you: your name, of course, but sometimes also your gender, your age, your implied ethnicity, and your circumstances (I have never mentioned a circumstantial detail that is uniquely yours). I will sometimes report something I heard you say within an episode from some other person's life. If you think you do see something personally recognisable in what I write, I can only apologise if you feel misused. In the appendix (p. 141-2) is a list of fifty characters, as I call them. The last person on the list, called Zola, is an emblem, concocted to make some theoretical points. The stories I tell about the others are all truthful, although not literally true.

Another point. I call you a patient at times when you are in relationship with a doctor, but not otherwise. People are patients when they are in a hospital, but not at home (usually). I sometimes call you 'my patient'. This is not because I imagine that I ever owned you, but you were mine at some point in the way that a shopkeeper's customers are his.

PART I

Illness

1

INTRODUCTION

Between Sickness and Health invites you to rethink illness. I write as a doctor and family therapist, but this book will not be a technical description of disease mechanisms or therapeutic remedies. I want to use what I know, along with whatever evidence can be found, to create a description of what it is to feel ill, and what it means to recover. I will be aspiring to see illness from a sufferer's rather than an observer's point of view. Such a picture becomes necessary when the concepts of illness and disease diverge, as they often do.

Illness is almost as unavoidable as being born, giving birth, growing, ageing and dying. A book about illness is therefore likely to touch on most aspects of what matters in human life. If this sounds excessively grand, think what happens when you are unwell. Anything from a humble cold to a mortal illness is liable to make you see your self and your life differently. You will also be seen differently by others; it is hard to be a serious person if you have a runny nose. When illness takes the lid off normality it exposes hopes and fears and social constraints – and even, occasionally, possibilities of liberation – that are invisible most of the time.

Writing the book has brought home to me that illness is not so much an aberration from normal life as an integral aspect of it. Illness creates culture. People who write or talk about their experiences of cancer, for example, are influencing contemporary attitudes towards life and death. Doctors such as myself are participants in the interpretation of the world, along with our patients. I should emphasise here that I am writing from within the 'Anglosphere', but the same dynamic relationship between illness and culture probably exists wherever people feel ill.

At one level, illness hardly seems to be a problem: isn't it just something to be endured where necessary and avoided if possible? And yet, the way we understand illness and its miseries makes a real difference to our lives. Ideas and feelings about illness directly affect the symptoms we experience and also shape the attitudes of the well towards the ill. Patients and doctors sometimes disagree about what should be counted as illness, and so do family members, friends, benefits assessors, therapists, teachers and others.[1] This book will 'erect signposts at all the junctions where there are wrong turnings so as to help people past the danger points'.[2] One wrong turning is to label someone's distress as medical without acknowledging its personal and social context. The danger here is of misconstruing the problem and hence seeking harmful or inadequate solutions. Explaining low mood in medical terms, for example, can sometimes be harmfully misleading, and so can treating obesity as an illness. An opposite wrong turning is to insist that someone who feels unwell is not really ill. The sufferings of people with psychiatric diagnoses are often dismissed as though they were not genuine illnesses, and those with contested conditions such as chronic fatigue syndrome or 'myalgic encephalomyelitis' (CFS/ME) often have the same experience.[3] Both these wrong turnings arise when illness is confused with disease. To be ill is to feel unwell, and I will be developing a concept of ill-being that encompasses all authentic feelings of illness, regardless of their biological or psychological basis.

Since illness is a feeling, what can be said, and who can say it? Social scientists write from a theoretical point of view about key themes such as culture, power and identity. Those with personal experience, on the other hand, write about what illness means in subjective terms. Clinicians such as myself are often positioned as objective observers, but at times our relationship with illness is highly personal so that we can form a useful bridge between experience and theory. I begin this introduction by explaining how my experiences as a doctor and family therapist have led to this book. I then outline the key themes and theoretical orientations, giving a selective overview of each chapter's themes.

I

When I was a medical student the primary object of study was not illness but disease.[4] I was taught to use clinical information mainly as a guide to diagnosis and at the bedside I was on the lookout for the patterns that diseases produce. A cough, a fever and a crackle in the lung suggested pneumonia, for example. We knew that breathlessness might be due to pneumonia, but if the ankles were swollen perhaps there was a problem with the heart. At that early stage I was too busy trying to make sense of what I could hear or see or smell to spare much thought for my patient's inner lives. Illness was a word for what you could see, not for what a person felt. Was the patient ill, or not? If so, how ill? This was an important question on an acute admission ward, where some patients needed urgent action while others could be left until later, or even dismissed. A patient who was 'genuinely ill', as we would put it, was someone with a definable disease. I had neither the time nor the incentive to discover what the symptoms of diseases felt like.

My years of specialist training in neurology were defined to a large extent by a distinction we were taught to make between real and unreal illness. When you are anxious it is easy to imagine you have multiple sclerosis (MS), because its sensory symptoms are very similar to the pins and needles and itches of normal life. Our patients often asked (as did the doctors who referred them) whether they were 'really ill'. What neurologists meant by the word anxiety was that the patient was not unwell. If you were anxious there was 'nothing wrong'.

Many people are immensely relieved to hear this, but it is hard to accept that you do not have an illness when you are convinced that you do. The most frustrating patients, for us, were the ones who claimed to be ill without any evidence of an 'organic' problem. Organic meant that an organ such as the brain or the heart was diseased. Complaints without an organic basis were (and often still are) called functional illness.[5] In their most extreme forms, they were diagnosed as hysterical conversion. This was a nod to Freud, who claimed that emotional disturbances could be converted into bodily forms, but the unvoiced assumption was that if an illness had an emotional basis it was not real.[6] On more than one occasion I heard David Marsden, the premier professor of neurology in our day, and a brilliant neuroscientist, refer to a person's functional symptoms as 'fake'. I was not happy with the supposed distinction between real and unreal illness, and my discomfort increased when I began meeting people diagnosed with CFS/ME. Symptoms such as fatigue, diffuse pain and lack of mental concentration produced real suffering, as anyone who lives or works with individuals will know, but the 'realness' of their symptoms cannot be confirmed objectively.

The nature of illness experience becomes hard to appreciate when it is defined by the image of disease as something visible and physical. This is just as true of organic as of functional conditions. During my specialist training I met people with Parkinson's disease who insisted that they were not ill but had every appearance of being so, particularly when responses to medication were erratic or inadequate. Their neurological impairments never went away, alas, and yet feelings of illness seemed to come and go. I began to realise that a doctor can no more determine whether a person is feeling ill than whether someone is or is not in pain.

Another crucial distinction I came across during my training was between illness and disability. Neurologists had even less interest in disability than in illness. Disability was something we trainees felt we should leave to occupational therapists and physiotherapists (which was another aspect of the way we were learning to keep our distance from our patients' personal experiences). I could not help getting interested in people's back-stories, however, once I began to 'follow' them in successive outpatient appointments as their neurological conditions progressed. They were continually bringing me questions about their practical lives. I was endlessly surprised by the effects of a condition such as Parkinson's disease on mobility, sleeping, thinking, sex and in fact every aspect of life. My patients were drawing me towards what I would now call their illness narratives. Patients' stories constantly suggested meanings that lay outside the narrow confines of a clinical history. Late in my medical career I discovered the value of exploring meanings through narratives without compromising the scientific approach to medicine, which I valued then, as I do now.

Narratives create a flow between different conceptions of illness. It suits the purposes of medicine to define illness in a certain way, but the experience of feeling ill is not well captured in biological language. Once free of its biomedical mould, however, illness becomes an ambiguous concept, threatening to fall apart entirely when we try to define it precisely. What exactly is the difference between disease and illness? What kinds of illness are real, and which are trivial? What do physical and mental illnesses have in common? Can illness have meanings? I quickly recognised as a doctor that addressing these questions requires a broader theoretical perspective than medicine can offer.

Anglo-American medical culture, in my experience, has a low opinion of theory. I remember a neurologist colleague beginning a lecture with a few tantalising remarks about the psychological causation of symptoms before cheerfully dismissing theory with a phrase I have often heard: 'Enough of philosophy!'. Doctors are so preoccupied with disease, as patients are with their sufferings, that theorising feels like a luxury. Theory is not a dull irrelevance to me, but a stimulus to the imagination. How else are we to be liberated from our prejudices? While I was a research registrar one of my patients presented me with a copy of Irving Goffman's sociological study of stigma.[7] He was inviting me to break through a barrier that divides practice from theory. This book extends the same invitation to clinicians and non-clinicians alike.

II

The theories needed in this book are not those of biology but of human life, as lived through personal narratives, because its purpose is to explore the meanings and implications of illness rather than the mechanics of disease. The book's clinical stories will mostly be connected with real people, but I want to begin by inventing one. Imagine two scenes in the life of a woman we'll call Zola. In Scene 1, Zola wakens in the middle of the night feeling 'off'. Being only half awake, she does not yet know what her offness is due to. It could be 'trouble, sorrow, need, sickness, or any other adversity'.[8] Zola is beginning to form the impression that she is ill. Switch to Scene 2. It's daytime, and Zola is on the phone to her employer, describing her unwellness. I am going to suggest some theoretical tools that help to make sense of these situations.

Contexts

One of the fundamentals in any approach to illness is the question of what counts as knowledge: this is what makes the issue of realness so painful for many people (Zola is forced to ask herself 'Am I really ill?'). Chapter 3, *Knowledges*, develops a contextual attitude to knowing realities such as illness, disease and disability. In Scene 1, Zola will draw on her common sense in order to make sense of her feelings. The anthropologist Clifford Geertz tells the story of a Zande potter who used his common sense to explain why one of his pots had cracked. He'd chosen the clay and worked it carefully, and he'd abstained from sexual intercourse the night before, so what else could it be but witchcraft?[9] Everyone's common-sense knowledge has a history and a sociology. Anthropologists and historians show how meanings arise from specific cultural contexts. What Zola comes to know about her experience will be influenced by the social and economic context in which she happens to live.

I am not decrying medical science, which has been my credo but, as RD Laing says, science must be adequate to its object. Biological science is less adequate than is social science, as a form of knowledge of illness experience; neither provide a full-blooded way of knowing human being. A 'science of persons', as Laing calls it,[10] must go further than either of these but it, too, must be constantly aware of context. Even such a common-sense notion as the body has a history[11].

Signs

A second fundamental is communication. The world's meanings are conveyed by signs. This is the starting point of Chapter 4, *Feelings*, where I explore what can be known of Zola's primary experience, its phenomenology. In Scene 2, Zola uses a culturally shared language of symptoms to establish a particular way of knowing what has happened to her.

Language is crucial in the field of illness because, as George Orwell tells us, it is an instrument not only for expressing things and but also for 'concealing or preventing thought'.[12] I will have something to say about the way the English language gives Zola a very questionable common-sense description of her illness as a concrete thing. Language is only part of the material from which illness is constructed. In Scene 2 she and someone else are in what Wittgenstein calls a language game. These very serious 'games' are not played solely in words; they consist of 'language and the actions into which it is woven'.[13] Bourdieu's sociological concept of habitus suggests that the body can convey meaning and produce knowledge independently of language. Actions can be 'reasonable without being the product of a reasoned design . . . intelligible and coherent without springing from an intention of coherence and a deliberate decision; adjusted to the future without being the product of a project or a plan'. What is learned, Bourdieu says, 'is not something that one has, like knowledge that can be brandished, but something that one is'.[14] Think of how Zola physically expresses her symptoms in Scene 2. In Chapter 5, *Appearances*, I describe the dramaturgical aspect of Scene 2 – the way in which Zola makes her feelings physically apparent to other people.

In writing this book I have become more aware that understandings and also misunderstandings of illness are often generated by pictures. As Wittgenstein said, pictures 'hold us captive'.[15] Pictures of disease are a dominant part of what Wittgenstein describes as 'the inherited background against which I distinguish between true and false'.[16] Illness tends to be assimilated into the disease picture so that it is difficult to see it in any other form. Pictures are profoundly influential in Scene 1 where Zola imagines what is wrong; also in medical diagnosis (Chapter 3); in the 'performance' of symptoms (Chapter 5); in exploring the meanings of illness (Chapter 6); and in concepts of wellness (Chapter 7).

Systems

Systems ideas provide an overarching approach in this book. The somewhat sterile-sounding concept of a system comes to life in Scene 2, where one person is talking to another, and where everything that is discussed is in relation to some other element within human and other systems. In Chapter 3 my contextual view derives from the assumption that knowledge is produced through the relational system that holds people together in their social world. The sociological perspectives that appear throughout this book always view social realities as being produced within human systems.

In Chapter 6, *Understandings*, a systemic perspective transcends both psychological and biological realms of explanation, because from a human point of view both are based on relationships between elements in systems. The physician and philosopher Georges Canguilhem rarely uses the word system but he conceives of illness in systemic terms, as a psychobiological transformation from one form of life to another.[17] I use the term interpretation to describe an approach to the understanding of illness as an experience, as distinct from the narrow sense of explanation as a linear chain of causes and effects. Elements within systems interact, so that what goes on is often the effect as well as the cause of something else that is happening. Merleau-Ponty says that the body creates meaning in the very process of expressing it: 'thought and expression . . . are simultaneously constituted, . . . as our body suddenly lends itself to some new gesture'.[18] In Scene 2 we can imagine how Zola's need to appear ill might have effects that will in turn affect how she feels.

Systems ideas have shown me how I, as a clinician, am placed within a therapeutic system. I will be offering a commentary on illness and medicine as an 'immanent' critic – one who is implicated in what I observe. I therefore cannot provide what Peter Sedgwick calls an 'exterior sociology'.[19]

Mind, body and self

Illness tends to turn difficult philosophical concepts into urgent personal questions. The problem of how to imagine the self rarely arises when we are well, but becomes a burning issue when illness disrupts a person's sense of integrity or continuity. Chapter 4 will argue that illness is a crisis of the self. Whatever conception we prefer, self is a way of summarising a central fact of personal life. Where else are we to locate pain, or death, if not in a self? Zola's ponderings in Scene 1 belong to a self. The body may vomit but it is the self that suffers. I do not see how this can be less true of someone whose culture has different conceptions of the self from mine.

The concept of mind is as much a pragmatic necessity in this book as is the language of self. The 'I' who is ill needs a locus other than the sick body, because otherwise there is no way of separating the self from the disease. However, we will see in subsequent chapters that thinking about illness undermines an absolute distinction between mind and body. Ill-being, as I conceive it, is a crisis of the body-self. I agree with Merleau-Ponty that 'there is not a word, not a form of behaviour which does not owe something to purely biological being – and which at the same time does not elude the simplicity of animal life'.[20]

Recovery

The book's last four chapters focus on routes towards recovery, which is viewed in a relative sense, as a process of orientation towards being 'better' at all stages in a person's living and dying. The concept of narrative becomes more prominent here. Narrative is a vehicle for meaning, although I have reservations about regarding illness either as a story or as a journey because these metaphors make illness sound more structured and more purposeful than it usually is.

In Chapter 7, *Possibilities*, I explore individuals' conceptions of wellness. I have in mind a framework that John Burnham recommends in systemic family therapy: 'Problems, possibilities, restraints and resources'.[21] I see recovery as a tendency, not an endpoint. Desire is a core concept here, and the locus of desire is the self. I begin with pictures and conceptions of health and well-being, and then turn to the personal forms of need that ill-being generates. I end with a description of the directions that people take in their pathways towards being 'better'.

Chapter 8, *Obstructions*, is about factors that obstruct the path towards recovery. Some biological obstacles are more or less immoveable. There are also sociological obstacles to recovery that are very hard for an individual to overcome, such as the role of health and social care systems in medicalising distress and in fostering or maintaining the status of illness. Other obstructions can be shifted: for example, one of the challenges of recovery is to leave a familiar way of life or an illness identity behind. This is difficult, but not impossible.

Chapter 9, *Resources*, turns to factors that promote recovery. Its starting point is not medical interventions but the elusive concept of healing. I review some non-medical resources that support healing and recovery, including places (for example hospitals and convalescent homes), regimens, and above all people. People provide interventions but their most vital roles in the promotion of healing include care, understanding and consolation.

Chapter 10, *Abilities*, returns to the personal perspective of Chapter 4. I suggest that resilience, a concept introduced in the previous chapter, need not be viewed as a set of innate traits or attitudes. A more hopeful view is that 'bouncing back' involves skills that can be developed.

Notes

1 In this book, 'patient' denotes someone who has a relationship with a doctor or other health professional. Not everyone who is ill is a patient, and nor are all patients ill.
2 Wittgenstein 1980, 18e
3 Ward 2015; Myalgic encephalomyelitis (ME) is a popular name based on a particular theory about the condition
4 See Atkinson 1997 for an account of how students' attitudes are formed during medical education
5 'Functional' and 'organic' disorders in the 19th century were those due, respectively, to physiological malfunctions or to a diseased organ. Neurologists often assume that 'functional' or 'non-organic' disorders are non-physical. The word functional survives in the DSM-5 (APA 2013) as an umbrella category. See www.neurosymptoms.org/
6 As a medical student I was startled when a physician, out of touch with his times, suggested the Freud-type diagnosis of 'rejection vomiting'
7 Goffman 1968
8 English Book of Common Prayer, 1662. http://justus.anglican.org/resources/bcp/
9 Geertz 1983 p. 78

10 Laing 1967, p. 17; 1960 Chapter 1
11 Smith 2017; Holmes 2010
12 Orwell 1946
13 Wittgenstein 1967 para 7
14 Bourdieu 1990 p. 50–51; 73
15 A picture held us captive, and we could not get outside it . . . Wittgenstein 1967, para 115; See Baker 2001, Patterson 2010. Wittgenstein 1977, para 94.
16 Wittgenstein 1977, para 94
17 Canguilhem 1991
18 Merleau-Ponty 2002 p. 207–213
19 Sedgwick 1982 p. 16 et seq.
20 Merleau-Ponty 2002 p. 220
21 See Burnham, J: https://bit.ly/2NlEHuA

2

IMAGES

Symptoms

- How are you? - Fine, fine. (I have tears unshed,
There is here near the bottom of my chest
a loop of cold, on the right.
A thing hurts somewhere up left in my head.
I have a gang of old sins unconfessed.
I shovel out of sight

a many-ills else…)
From 'Dreamsong 207'. John Berryman[1]

The abyss

There is a pain—so utter—
It swallows substance up—
Then covers the Abyss with Trance—
So Memory can step
Around—across—upon it—
As one within a Swoon—
Goes safely—where an open eye—
Would drop Him—Bone by Bone.
Emily Dickinson[2]

She lay on a narrow ledge over a pit that she knew to be bottomless, though she
could not comprehend it; the ledge was her childhood dream of danger, and she
strained back against a reassuring wall of granite at her shoulders, staring into the
pit, thinking, There it is, there it is at last, it is very simple; and soft carefully
shaped words like oblivion and eternity are curtains hung before nothing at all.
Katherine Anne Porter[3]

Struggle

The worse her condition grew, the more she bent all her thoughts and all her energies
upon her illness, for which she felt a naïve hatred. Nearly all her life she had been a

woman of the world, with a quiet, native, and permanent love of life and good living. . . But the gentle death was not to be hers.

Thomas Mann[4]

Transformation

[In illness] we cease to be soldiers in the army of the upright; we become deserters. They march to battle. We float with the sticks on the stream; helter-skelter with the dead leaves on the lawn, irresponsible and disinterested and able, perhaps for the first time for years, to look 'round, to look up—to look, for example, at the sky.'

Virginia Woolf. On Being Ill[5]

Teach us to out to outgrow our madness

Her tears stirred an echo in my troubled and suffering heart; I forgot my illness and everything else in the world; I walked about the drawing-room and muttered distractedly . . .

Anton Chekhov. Anonymous story[6]

Metaphors

And then, as the other world produces serpents and vipers, malignant and venomous creatures, and worms and caterpillars, that endeavour to devour that world which produces them, and monsters compiled and complicated of divers parents and kinds; so this world, ourselves, produces all these in us, in producing diseases, and sicknesses of all those sorts: venomous and infectious diseases, feeding and consuming diseases, and manifold and entangled diseases made up of many several ones.

John Donne[7]

Care

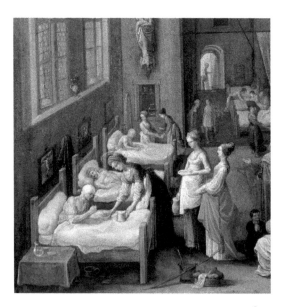

FIGURE 2.1 St Elizabeth visiting a hospital. Adam Elsheimer 1598.[8]

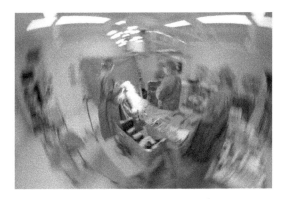

FIGURE 2.2 Hospital operating theatre, UK. Adrian Wressell.[9]

Convalescence

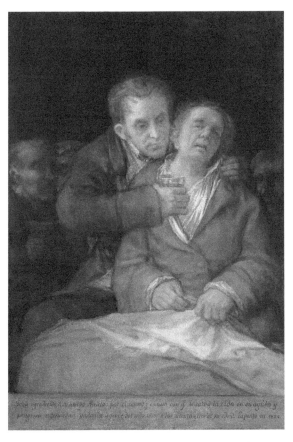

FIGURE 2.3 Self-portrait with Dr Arrieta. Francisco Goya, 1820[10]

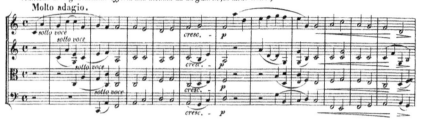

FIGURE 2.4 Ludwig van Beethoven (Holy Song of Thanks by a Convalescent to the Deity).[11]

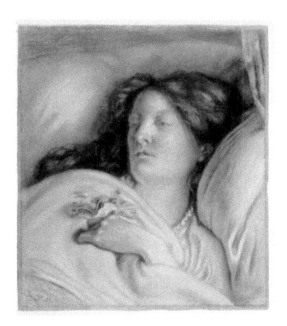

FIGURE 2.5 Convalescent. Ford Madox Brown 1872.[12]

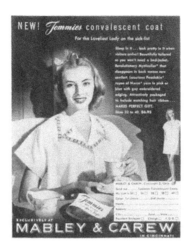

FIGURE 2.6 Tommies convalescent coat. For the loveliest lady on the sick list. *The Ladies' Home Journal* 1948.[13]

Convalescence

First you must find a view,
then make a quilt of get well cards
and good wishes. Then unravel yourself,
each knot and tangle, crease and fist.
Undo them. Listen to each limb and crevice,
the voices of your bones,
chart the weather of your body,
the nuances of each breath.
Eat the food of your childhood,
Haliborange and small fingers of bread.
Wear dirty slippers. Forget about words

and pay particular attention to trees.
Be wary of animals and children.
Play Gregorian chants. No mirrors.
Do not wash. Watch insects.
Let things roll under the bed.
Do not plan. Remove all diaries
Be weak. Be languid.
Flow back into yourself
slowly, tentatively,
when the dust has settled
on the windowsill,
and you have quite forgotten
the colour of work.

Julia Darling 2003[14]

Dying

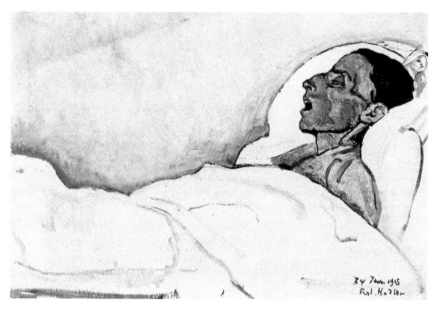

FIGURE 2.7 Valentine Godé-Darel one day before her death. Ferdinand Hodler 1915.[15]

Notes

1 The opening lines of Dreamsong 207, from John Berryman. *Dreamsongs*. Farrar, Straus and Giroux, 1969. By kind permission of the publishers.
2 There is a pain – so utter . . . Emily Dickinson. Written 1862, published 1929. The last two lines in the handwritten version contain alternatives: Goes *steady* —where an open eye— Would *spill* Him — Bone by Bone
3 Katherine Anne Porter. *Pale Horse Pale Rider*, Harcourt, Brace 1939
4 Thomas Mann. *Buddenbrooks*. Translated from the German by H.T. Lowe-Porter. London Martin Secker, 1922. Part 9, Chapter 1
5 Virginia Woolf. *On Being Ill*. 1926
6 Anton Chekhov, A (1893). 'An anonymous story'. Transl. C Garnett: In: *The Lady with the Dog and Other Stories*, 1917
7 John Donne. Meditation IV, Devotions Upon Emergent Occasions, and severall steps in my Sicknes, 1624
8 St Elizabeth visiting a hospital. Adam Elsheimer. 1598. Wellcome Collection
9 Hospital operating theatre UK. Adrian Wressell. Wellcome Collection
10 Goya's depiction of himself in critical illness was painted in gratitude to his physician friend Dr Arrieta. Minneapolis Institute of Art, Minnesota.
11 Opening bars of 3rd movement, Quartet Op 132, Beethoven, Ludwig van Beethoven
12 Ford Madox Brown. Convalescent. Portrait of Emma Madox Brown. 1872. Birmingham Museum and Art Gallery

13 Tommies' Convalescent Coat, Mabley & Carew. *Ladies Home Journal* 1889. Internet Archive Book Images.
14 Julia Darling. Convalescence. From: *Sudden Collapses in Public Places*. Todmorden, Lancashire: Arc Publications, 2003. Reproduced by kind permission of the publishers.
15 Ferdinand Hodler Valentine Godé-Darel one day before her death. 1915. Kunstmuseum Basel.

3

KNOWLEDGES

Illness is a feeling. The next chapter looks at symptoms from the inside, but I want to begin here with the question of how feelings can become known as illness. Within the domain of medicine knowledge appears to be continually reaching towards completion. This triumphalist view misrepresents the nature of both medicine and knowledge. Knowledge has a history and a sociology, just as medicine does. What counts as true is influenced by the social, economic and intellectual worlds we live in.[1] Jewson describes medical 'cosmologies' that 'prescribe the visible and the invisible, the imaginable and the unimaginable'.[2] In a neuroscience-determined cosmology, what is imaginable often conjures up the image of an MR scan. One of the aims in this chapter is to show that dominant constructs of our Western cosmology such as diagnosis, disease and disability render some aspects of illness almost unimaginable.

Think again of Zola from Chapter 1, with her feelings of unwellness. Imagine she is suffering from fatigue and bodily aches. She lives on her own and has neither the energy nor the appetite to eat well at the moment. She's been dragging herself to work but is on the brink of resigning. What she knows for sure is that she is not herself. Her mother died a year ago, but nothing else has gone wrong in her life. She is looking for a way of understanding her feelings: a way of knowing them.

If we want to understand the experience of Zola or any ill person, biological facts are not the central issue. A medical text can describe 'what is known' about Zola's experience but I want to ask how she comes to know it as illness, regardless of whether anyone else would know it in the same way. Her ways of knowing derive from her various relationships with the world.

Illness is an episode in Zola's social life, and therefore a piece of sociology. The way she sees her troubles is inseparable from her cultural context, which gives illness an anthropology. Zola very likely inhabits more than one culture: her symptoms might derive their meanings from her knowledge of orthodox medicine, from ideas that her mother gave her as a child, from her religious background, if she has one, and from any number of other sources. There is no single, canonical body of facts about illness. There are knowledges.

Classification

Language sorts experience into categories.[3] Medical diagnosis is one version of the human tendency, or need, to categorise people. Social life depends on categorical thinking. Feelings receive labels such as 'embarrassment', 'panic' and 'grief'. From a social point of view each of these is a diagnosis. A journalist musing on the poet Emily Dickinson offers diagnoses of these kinds: 'What was going on? It's all too tempting to speculate . . . Did she suffer from acute social anxiety, or epilepsy, or bipolar disorder? Was she a lesbian, a proto-feminist, a religious radical, a sexual pioneer?'[4]

Being categorised is an uncomfortable experience. TS Eliot writes of 'the eyes that fix you in a formulated phrase' leaving you 'sprawling on a pin'. You would get the feeling of being pinned down even if you were given a spurious label such as 'gazebism' or 'garrutopia' or 'Crystal's syndrome' (I made these ones up – but see Wikipedia's list of fictional diseases). The authority of a diagnosis arises partly from its grammar.[5] 'The' diagnosis suggests something concrete and definite, so that we wonder if Zola has 'got' chronic fatigue syndrome[6] (or maybe Crystal's syndrome?).[7] A diagnosis, like an illness, represents something abnormal; it is generally something unwelcome.[8] Another key point is that a medical diagnosis always belongs to just one person: Zola necessarily 'has' her own diagnosis or illness, even if her distress is something shared.[9] The grammar that makes diagnosis a thing leads us, in Western culture at any rate, to expect an explanation for 'it', because every object in the universe sits somewhere along a chain of causes and effects. A diagnosis may make it seem as though everything Emily Dickinson did or said could be explained in some single way.

Giving someone a medical diagnosis frames specific aspects of the person as medical knowledge. It is never certain who will get swept up in a classificatory net and who will escape, because categories of medical knowledge are constantly changing.[10] Even the most implausible of diagnoses can catch on. A notorious example is 'drapetomania', which was supposed to 'explain' a slave's pathological wish to escape. Drapetomania did not last long, thankfully. Diagnoses often become obsolete. Less contentious labels than drapetomania, for example bronchitis and rheumatism, have been edged out of medical orthodoxy over time. Repetitive strain injury come to social prominence for a while and then fade away. The names used for depression have varied throughout the last 50 years, reflecting the changing context of psychiatry over that period[11]. On the whole, more diagnoses are born than die. The American Psychiatry Association's Diagnostic and Statistical Manual (DSM) has expanded its list of diagnoses in successive editions. Some diagnoses are waiting in the wings. 'Pervasive refusal syndrome' is described in one mainstream medical journal as life-threatening, but it has yet to get into the DSM. There is constant pressure to split existing diagnoses into still more categories; there is said to be a

'need for subtypes' in chronic fatigue syndrome; and 'pathological demand avoidance' has been described as 'a necessary distinction' among neurodevelopmental
disorders such as autism. Certain social situations seem close to being incorporated
into the medical way of knowing, for example 'anxious school refusal', and so do
certain moods.[12] I wonder if boredom might one day become a diagnosis in the
International Classification of Diseases. Shyness has already been medicalised,
according to one critic.[13]

   Any doctor who has tried to explain to an ill patient precisely what is going on, or
any worker who has 'phoned in sick' will sometimes have longed for a simple label
rather than having to shoulder the burden of explanation. 'It's a stroke' or 'it's flu'
might be enough. The power of a diagnosis to simplify can be destructive, however.
If you are in despair, it might be worse than useless to be told 'you've got depression'. The historian Jacob Burckhardt coined the term 'terrible simplificateur', or
terrible simplification, to describe an account of a situation that 'denies the existence
of anything more complicated than itself'.[14] Even the most authentic of clinical
diagnoses can do this, as when the label 'Alzheimer's disease' is assumed to explain
everything that the affected person feels or thinks or does. When a complex phenomenon, for example obesity, is transformed into a medical diagnosis, an aspect of
the problem such as economic deprivation may become invisible. Someone who is
left sprawling on a pin, like a lepidopterist's butterfly, has become a mere type rather
than an individual, which was why we medical students too often slipped into
speaking of someone as 'the heart failure in bed ten'.

   The ideal definition of a category is conjunctive, or monothetic. A conjunctive
approach lists all the features distinguishing it from any other category.[15] We
should not be surprised that this is rarely possible in medicine, because it is hard
to make a conjunctive definition even of a chair. Most properties of a chair are
shared by other objects such as sofas and stools and even tables. We mostly use a
disjunctive (or polythetic) method to classify things, identifying them by what
Wittgenstein called family resemblances.[16] A horse has four legs, but so does a
chair; it neighs, but so does a zebra, and yet family resemblances distinguish
chairs, zebras and horses. Although measles always involves the measles virus,
most of its manifestations can either be present or absent in individual cases.
Depression reduces your appetite but so does anxiety; it may either make you
sleepy or keep you awake; it can make you look sad, but not in every case. Major
depression, according to the latest edition of the DSM (DSM-5) requires you to
have five from a list of eight symptoms, including at least one of the first two.
Two people meeting the same criteria could each have a different principal
symptom and only two symptoms in common. CFS/ME is diagnosed, according to
a widely-used scheme, if there is fatigue plus four of eight symptoms, so that two
people with the same diagnosis might have only fatigue in common. Neurasthenia,
CFS/ME's cousin, can be diagnosed in the International Classification of Diseases
without fatigue, which shows how family resemblances can drift away from their
'centre of variation'.[17] The kind of knowledge that disjunctive definitions produces is
far from solid.

Many diagnoses are over-used, but they do help to identify different kinds of distress. The profile called depression, for example, is recognisable, and different from the one that psychiatrists call mania. Labels such as obsession compulsion disorder (OCD) and attention deficit hyperactivity disorder (ADHD) may be applied too often but they do describe patterns that occur in groups of real people; so also do equally over-used medical labels such as flu, ME and osteoarthritis. There are times when a label points towards a plan of action that would not otherwise be visible. The diagnosis of depression, people often complain, is an excuse for excessive medication and ECT, but labelling someone as depressed does alert us to the risk of suicide and the need for care.

The idea of illness

Illness is difficult to define. A first step is to distinguish it from disease. Disease is 'a disorder of structure or function in a human, animal, or plant'.[18] The disorders that diseases produce are called impairments[19], and impairments can always be observed by one means or another. Limb impairments are visible to the naked eye, but renal impairments only become visible through chemical tests.

In everyday language, the idea of disease absorbs that of illness as though there was no difference between them. One online definition defines disease as 'an *illness* of people, animals, plants, etc. caused by infection or a failure of health'[20], but there is something wrong with treating disease and illness as synonyms. We can surely have disease without illness. Athlete's foot and dental caries are diseases, but they do not make us feel ill. We can also have illness without disease. Morning sickness in pregnancy might make you feel very ill, but it is not a disease. The illness suffered by people diagnosed with CFS/ME can be debilitating but there is barely a shred of evidence for any disease process.[21] No-one who has been severely depressed, or who has been close to such a person (as I have), will quarrel with the word illness, but depression is not a disease like malaria or cancer.

Unlike disease, illness is often invisible. We cannot see depression. Agonising back pain or chaotic bowel disturbances or crippling fatigue or severe anxiety can occur without any observable 'disorder of structure and function'. Back pain triggers muscle spasms and anxiety alters the heart rate, but these are appropriate physiological responses. They are effects rather than causes. It is always possible to say that illness is caused by a disease that we cannot yet see, but we will never be able to see depression, or anxiety, or pain, or fatigue until we can read each others' minds[22]. Of all the troubles that Zola reports the one that is most definitive of illness, I suggest, is that she does not feel 'herself', which is not something that can be proved with a brain scan or a blood test.

I want to reserve the idea of illness for something that grasshoppers, snakes and elm trees do not experience; reptiles and insects have feelings, and perhaps even trees do, but they do not feel ill. They have diseases, but illness is a subjective reality that only humans know about. The word illness gives Zola a particular, culturally-determined way of knowing her feelings, which makes it a useful social construct. Christopher Boorse somewhere wrote that we do not regard a diseased fruit-fly as ill for much the same reason that we do not feel the need to give it a decent funeral. Human culture determines who gets a funeral. People perform burial ceremonies for animals they choose to think of as honorary persons, including horses, cats, dogs and budgies, but not usually pigs or chickens.[23]

Illness is a construct, not a chimera. Medicine and medical language will determine what will or will not count as illness, but medicine owes its existence to the fact that people do feel ill. Every culture, so far as I know, has produced medical, magical and religious healers. They are not a response to disease but to a species of felt need that we call illness.[24] I will be using the notion of ill-being to identify feelings of need that head in the direction of a medical account without necessarily being confined to it.

Ways of knowing and ways of not-knowing

Imagine Zola feeling 'off' (corresponding to Scene 1 in Chapter 1). She is exhausted and has a splitting headache, and is talking to her friend Anna about her feelings (Scene 2). Figure 3.1 roughly represents the raw materials for a dialogue about feelings of unwellness. I will explore the feelings themselves in the next chapter. The question here is how they come to be known as illness.

Constructing illness

There is a two-way relationship between how a person thinks about unwellness and how she experiences it. Her distress will mean one thing if she concludes she is ill and another if she attributes it to something else. Until Zola is sure she is ill her feelings will defy interpretation, and yet she does know that her usual sense of wellness has evaporated and that a new form of life has taken over. This is Zola's personal knowledge,[25] and I think such knowledge is undeniable even if it cannot be verified scientifically. Who else can say that a person is or is not herself?

Zola's problem is that the world uses its own criteria to distinguish the sick from the well, the abnormal from the normal, the genuine from the fake. How can her personal knowledge of unwellness be converted into common knowledge? How can it be aligned with the way Anna, or her employer or her doctor see things? How can she be accepted as 'genuine'? She cannot simply say 'I don't feel myself', or 'please, boss, give me a break'. Zola can hardly avoid using illness language, which is one of the few culturally sanctioned ways of knowing human distress. And illness language, in the public sphere, condenses into a diagnosis that almost inevitably implies disease.

Once Zola steps into 'the kingdom of the sick'[26] she and Anna will find it possible to draw on conventional constructs such as symptoms, illness, disease, diagnosis, and so on. We cannot make personal experience intelligible to others without constructs. The construct of illness is not so much a coherent description as a habitus, in Bourdieu's sense[27], that organises feelings, thoughts and behaviours. This is how Zola has acquired the ability to perform her suffering in a way that makes it credible to her friend Anna. Their common sense enables them to obey the rules of a medical language game together. They are given a 'way of knowing' Zola's distress, even though there might be alternative, non-medical ways of responding to it.

Zola and Anna are not simply construction workers on a cultural production line, however. Their dialogue is more fluid and more dynamic than that. When Zola says 'Maybe I'm ill' she forms a link in what Mikhail Bakhtin describes as a 'chain of speech communion', setting off 'dialogical reverberations'[28] that resonate with previous conversations. What comes to Zola and Anna may be pictures rather than words. For me, the notion of illness conjures up images, sounds and smells that go back to childhood. We have a sort of visceral knowledge of what it is to feel ill. I say 'we' tentatively. I hope that this book will be in dialogue with readers whose cultural milieux that are outside my experience. There are different knowledges because there are different common senses.[29] There would no doubt be important differences between Ugandan nuns, Russian oligarchs and Fiji farmers in how they communicated distress to one another.

In this book we are at least as interested in Zola's experience as we are in her social context. An important question for us is how well the cultural apparatus of illness serves Zola's efforts to understand and communicate her distress. Language is a constraint, because the way we imagine illness is so much influenced by the words we use. Grammar will inevitably make it seem as though Zola has an illness in the same way that she has a pair of kidneys. George Orwell said that language corrupts thought,[30] which it certainly does when it forces feelings of illness into a concrete mould. The grammar of things will prompt Zola herself, as well as her friend and everyone she meets, to ask thing-based questions. What is it? What will it do to you? How can you I rid of it? These are not the right questions for every kind of distress. Feeling states can belong to 'the turbid ebb and flow of human misery'[31] without representing anything concrete. They tend to get swamped by the idea of disease.

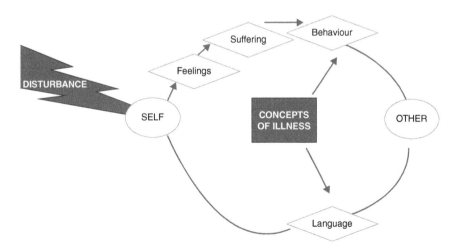

FIGURE 3.1 Dialogue converts feeling into an illness

Disease: entity or system?

Disease evokes pictures. Perhaps we imagine blotchy skin, or an emaciated body, or death. Pestilence is one of the four horses of the apocalypse, and we think of disease as something we 'get' from the outside.[32] But disease is not a free-standing entity that stalks the world in search of trouble. It is a system, like any other. A system is any 'set of elements standing in relation among themselves and with the environment'.[33] The brain is a system of neurons; the body is a system of systems; and a disease is also a system. Osteoarthritis, for example, is a system that relates genes, joint surfaces and mechanical stresses, among other things, just as rust is a system that relates metal, oxygen and water. Infections are no different. Poliomyelitis is a system that includes viruses, target tissues (motor neurons) and the immune system.

What a system looks like is a question of perspective. Mouldy food is bad, but mouldy blue cheese is good. Polio infection is a disaster for a human but for a virus it is all in a day's work. This is what Epictetus means when he says that a fever is a part of life like a stroll, a voyage, a journey.[34] Ivan Illich makes the same melancholy point: 'Man's consciously lived fragility, individuality, and relatedness make the experience of pain, of sickness, and of death an integral part of his life'.[35] We shift from one perspective to another by 'punctuating' the systemic phenomenon of disease in different ways.[36]

Symptoms can often be punctuated as processes of repair rather than destruction. In osteoarthritis, deformities of spinal and limb joints are produced through the tendency for damaged bone and cartilage to replace itself. Any immune reaction is an attempt to protect the body, even though it may be destructive rather than helpful. The 17th century physician Thomas Sydenham wrote that 'a disease, however much its cause may be adverse to the human body, is nothing more than an effort of Nature, who strives with might and main to restore the health of the body'.[37] Sydenham's essentially systemic picture of disease can be traced to the Hippocratic physicians of ancient Greece. Modern concepts of physiological regulation are a scientific equivalent of the humoral balance that Hippocratic doctors described. Equilibrium is maintained in a physiological system by homeostasis. In illness the system becomes unstable and is transformed, although biological systems can settle into a new equilibrium through a process that has been called allostasis.[38]

Disease, like illness, is a construct that involves punctuating processes in a particular way. It is a myth - not a falsehood, but a story that generates particular meanings. For many people the disease myth carries all before it. They imagine that disease is something 'mankind' can ultimately conquer.[39] Sir Richard Quain, a late Victorian doctor, declared that since 'physiology has in recent days diffused a clear and penetrating light over the many of the processes of life in health' it should soon be possible to supply a precise definition of 'what disease really is'.[40]

Punctuating disease as a concrete entity provides a way of knowing illness and at the same time a very specific way of not knowing.[41] Sir Richard Quain assumes that any deviation from wellness should have a biological explanation. A scientist in our own times, no less up-beat than Sir Richard, asserts that 'we do not know the cause of chronic fatigue syndrome, or ME, for the same reason that we do not know the cause of many neurologic diseases: we have not yet been clever enough to figure it out'.[42] The implication is that feelings of illness must refer to a disease of some sort. Insisting on a 'distinction between the world of physical objects and mental states' is what the anthropologist Byron Good calls medical objectivism.[43] According to this way of thinking, any genuine symptom must have a physical rather than a merely psychological or social explanation. Another confident Victorian doctor expresses the objectivist point of view bluntly: 'Medical men deal not with words but with things'.[44] I agree with Good that in some situations, for example in CFS/ME, or in Zola's medically unexplained pain, or in depression, objectivism 'so obscures understanding as to render the phenomenon largely unintelligible'.

Normality

Nothing exposes the tension between subjective and objective conceptions of illness more completely than the idea of normality. To feel ill is to feel bad, but what counts as bad? There are various species of normality, each with its own effects on the way we think about illness.

Bodily impairment

For a medical objectivist, 'wrongness' always means biological abnormality. An adult heart that cannot pump out five or so litres of blood every minute is abnormal, as is a brain that cannot add up. Measuring an organ's physical functions detects disease, but it is not a realistic way of gauging the impact of illness or injury on an individual. Twice as much physical impairment could produce four times as much misery in some situations, but it might make only a small difference in others. Nonetheless miners receive compensation for lung disease in proportion to what percentage of normal lung function they have lost. The Department of Health and Social Service (DHSS) used to take the view that a person who was missing one leg was 25% disabled, a logic that could have absurd results.

The degree of impairment does not predict distress very well. In the first place, the body's reserve capacities often cushion us from relatively minor injuries. We do have pairs of eyes and ears and kidneys, and even the brain has some adaptive capacity. Secondly, there are biological, psychological and social reasons why a given disorder of structure and function has a much bigger impact on some individuals than on others. Taste and smell, for example, are not equally important to everyone. One young kitchen assistant did not know he had lost his sense of smell until someone else noticed that the stew he was stirring smelt terrible. If we want to understand an impaired individual's overall experience, we need to take that person's daily existence into account.

Incapacity

Life depends to a great degree on what a person can do, so that incapacity might get closer than impairment to defining the feeling of 'wrongness' or abnormality that illness produces. If your eyes are impaired but you wear glasses, your capacity to see things may be good enough for your purposes. Zola's capacities can be compared to those that adults like her are expected to have, such as walking and talking. The World Health Organization (WHO)'s original list of capacities called them disabilities, later changed to activity limitations.[45] I was often asked to complete a form for people seeking state benefits. One of the questions concerned the patient's ability to climb a ladder (I did my best to answer this, although there was never a ladder to hand in the clinic). The assumption that a person's productivity could be determined normatively was flawed. Zola very probably could climb down or up a ladder if her house was on fire, which would say nothing about the impact of illness on her life.

It is important to be clear here that incapacity is not illness. Someone whose legs have been amputated is neither more nor less likely to feel ill than anyone else. Incapacity is not illness, but on the other hand illness is always, in a sense, incapacity. If I say 'I am not myself today' I am reporting a personal incapacity: I feel less able to be the person I think I am, or to lead the life I think I should. Social norms cannot fully define this kind of incapacity.

Injustice

Incapacities reduce a person's chances of enjoying the same quality of life as someone with average abilities. The WHO described such disadvantages originally as handicaps and subsequently as restrictions in participation. The inability to walk up a flight of stairs produces obvious disadvantages. Impairments in vision, hearing or cognition are less visible but equally restrictive. Illness can also produce incapacities that are not due to an impairment, i.e. not attributable to a disorder of bodily structure or function. The stigma of a psychiatric diagnosis, for example, can seriously reduce the possibility of leading one's chosen life.

It is clearly unfair that someone's life should be restricted by something as arbitrary and oppressive as stigma, and the same assumption extends to more obvious disadvantages such as the inaccessibility of buildings to people in wheelchairs. The normative principle in all these situations is justice.

Imbalance

We have an intuition, too complex philosophically to explore here, that fairness is the way things ought naturally to be. A more general intuition defines what is bad or good in terms of what is unnatural. Georges Canguilhem pointed out that only organisms have pathologies. There is no such thing as a pathological hammer or a pathological volcano, because such things are always in a state that is natural to them. Pathology is a word for the state that an organism gets into when its normal way of existing is in some way interrupted. We think of illness as unnatural because we punctuate it as a deviation from the way a person (as distinct from an inanimate object, or even an objectified body) ought to be. We hope for a return to some kind of balance, or equilibrium, or harmony.

Personal 'wrongness'

Zola may have all the physiological functions and capacities the WHO lists and yet not be able to be her normal self. My clinical experience brought me into contact with many patients who failed objective tests of illness and yet were manifestly ill, and clearly suffering. They were adrift from their own normalities, if not from medicine's. The psychiatrist Jerome Wakefield argues that mental illness is 'harmful dysfunction'. Harm connects with personal meanings and values, while dysfunction is what makes mental illness factually different from other negative conditions such as ignorance and criminality.[46] However, function is not a purely objective, factual issue. It involves values when it makes assumptions about what a person is for. A person's objective capacities are only a part of what we are thinking of when we notice that an ill person is not functioning properly.

I will explore the quality of illness experience in the next chapter. My question here is what Zola means when she says she knows she feels wrong. What she can share with others is a sense of badness. The Greek root kak- covers not only illness but also badness generally, as well as evil. The French mal generates maladie, meaning both illness and disease, but it amounts to an aesthetic judgement across the series of translations that one website offers; not only ailment, pain, ache, hurt and harm, but also bad, wrong, poorly, difficult, trouble, hard time, insufficiently, mischief, rot.[47] These judgements of badness are not physiological, or practical, but aesthetic. It might seem odd, if not offensive, to speak of medicine and aesthetics in the same breath.[48] The only people who routinely do so are cosmetic surgeons and orthodontists, for whom aesthetics means beauty. However, the worst of experiences, as well as the best, produce aesthetic reactions. In English, the word 'ill' overlaps with judgements we could certainly call aesthetic (ill-fitting, ill-suited, etc). Physical, moral and aesthetic offences to a person's sense of what is natural and good find their way into the meaning of illness (Chapter 6), and hence of wellness (Chapter 7).

Towards a different way of knowing and not-knowing illness

'To be sick', according to Canguilhem, 'means that a person really leads another life, even in the biological sense of the word'.[49] Canguilhem's essentially systemic perspective blurs distinctions between illness and disease, and also between mind and body, so that it becomes possible to think of all forms of illness in both physical and non-physical terms.

The 'other life' of illness brings about a 'transformation of the sick person's personality', and hence belongs to an individual rather than to a class of persons who share the same diagnosis.[50] The emerging field of personalised medicine mirrors this insight in its focus on genes and other characteristics that are unique to individuals.[51] No two cases of cancer, or epilepsy, or CFS/ME, or depression are identical. One biologist suggests that 'what we have in common as members of a single species is not so much a set of specific, fixed characteristics as a set of flexible biological responses'. He says that 'culture and society play a formative part in shaping the context in which these [biological] responses occur'.[52] There are sets of flexible psychological and social responses as well as biological ones, and illness experiences are an amalgam of all of three. These responses produce recognisable patterns such as immune responses and stress reactions that are 'final common pathways' in illness.[53] A diagnosis is a useful way of summarising a pattern but can be a terrible simplification that is liable to promote specious medical explanations for the 'other life' of illness.

Medicalisation is an arbitrary process 'by which nonmedical problems become defined and treated as medical problems'. As a result, 'differences in learning styles become learning disabilities or ADHD; divergences in sexual desires or performance become sexual dysfunctions; extremes of behavior become sexual, shopping, or internet addiction . . . ; and individual differences become . . . social phobia'.[54] But how are human troubles to be understood if not as illness, and how are unhappy people are to be helped if not by doctors? One critic of medicalisation looks back to a time when 'a myriad virtues . . . traditionally enabled people to recognise painful sensations as a challenge and to shape their own experience accordingly'.[55] This romantic picture is historically naïve. In traditional as well as modern societies, medicine has always been a resource for people who feel ill, aiming to provide interventions that help them feel better. Rather than calling for medicine to dismantle itself, a more realistic objective will be to remind doctors to respond to illness as something distinct from disease.

Notes

1 See Burke 2012, for the sociology of knowledge and especially Chapter 5 for a description of how knowledge ebbs as well as flows through history. See Pickstone 2000 for an account of different 'ways of knowing' in the history of medicine
2 Jewson 1976
3 See McHugh and Slavney 1986 on this point, and for an excellent discussion of the issues raised by medical diagnosis
4 William Nicholson. Guardian 1/4/17
5 TS Eliot, The Love Song of J. Alfred Prufrock, 1917; https://en.wikipedia.org/wiki/List_of_fictional_diseases; see Ward 2015 c– 'What does the diagnosis say?'
6 The diagnosis of CFS/ME applies to people who are undoubtedly ill, sometimes severely so, but there is no evidence for a disease that causes their symptoms. In our book *Meanings of ME* (Ward 2015) we strove to use language that left open the question of whether CFS/ME was itself an entity. I never made CFS/ME the subject of a sentence, and I referred to 'people diagnosed with CFS/ME' in an effort not to ether assert

or deny that CFS/ME was an autonomous 'thing'. The moment I relaxed my guard the concrete grammar of illness crept in

7 A syndrome is a collection of things that often occur together, and so need not be a thing at all. Wikipedia lists 1429 medical syndromes

8 Names have a peculiar mystique, however, and there are those who would be glad to have the rare (in fact unique) diagnosis of garrutopia. ('There is a small dose of revenge in every complaint' Nietzsche – *The Twilight of the Idols*)

9 It is possible that some of these properties of a diagnosis reflect a culture in which ownership and private property are valued. Might medical labels distribute themselves differently in a culture where things are not seen as 'belongings'?

10 One source of confusion arises between criteria used for practical diagnosis and the narrower criteria that are used in clinical research. For an example in joint disease see Aggarwal et al. 2015

11 Pickstone 2000

12 Drapetomania – Cartwright 1851; repetitive strain – MacEachen 2005; depression – McPerson & Armstrong 2006; pervasive refusal syndrome – Lask 2004; chronic fatigue syndrome – Jason et al. 2005; pathological demand avoidance – Newson et al. 2003

13 Since writing this I have found Burgler (1945) On the Disease-entity Boredom 'Alysosis' and its Psychopathology; see Scott 2006 on the medicalisation of shyness

14 See Watzlawick et al. 1974 Chapter 4

15 See McHugh & Slavney 1986 p. 26–31; Adams et al. 2002

16 Wittgenstein 1967; see also Barraclough 2004 for a view on Wittgenstein's earlier and later ideas about language, in relation to diagnosis

17 DSM – APA 2013; neurasthenia WHO (2016), ICD-10, F-48; centre of variation – another concept from Wittgenstein, see Baker 2001

18 Oxford Dictionaries online

19 WHO 2001

20 Cambridge Dictionaries online

21 See Ward 2015 a

22 See Chapter 6 for more on yet-to-be-discovered diseases

23 I leave open the question of animal culture. See De Waal 2001

24 Peter Sedgwick, no friend of positivist medical science, makes this point well (1982, p. 32) although he does not clearly distinguish illness from disease

25 See Polanyi 1958. 'I regard knowing as an active comprehension of the things known, an action that requires skill'

26 Sontag 1978

27 Habitus: see Chapter 1

28 Bakhtin 1986, p. 84; p. 94

29 Common sense as described by Geertz 1983, p. 78

30 Orwell 1946

31 Matthew Arnold. Dover Beach, 1867

32 It is easy to see why people prefer the label 'Parkinson's' or 'Huntington's', rather than attaching the word 'disease' to those diagnoses

33 See: www.panarchy.org/vonbertalanffy/systems.1968.html. Also, Von Bertalanffy 1972; Boulding 1956

34 Epictetus (2nd century CE/1956) Book 3, Chapter 10 v.11

35 Illich 1976, p. 275

36 See Chapter 1. For an accessible history of this concept see Guillermo 1980. I watched a confused woman being coaxed by two nurses to take a tablet that was balanced precariously on her tongue. Eventually she said 'Sorry sister. I've swallowed it'. Here were two incompatible punctuations of the same 'offer-accept' loop

37 Sydenham 1665. Sydenham is associated with the idea of disease as an entity (an 'ontological' as opposed to a physiological concept – see Temkin 1963), but here he depicts a physiological or systemic process

38 See Ramsay and Woods 2014; Modell et al. 2015

39 Porter 1997 *The Greatest Benefit to Mankind*. The phrase is from Samuel Johnson's life of Dr Herman Boerhaave, 1739 (he considered the medical profession the second greatest benefit to mankind)

40 Quain 1895 – 'Disease'

41 See Ward 2015d – 'So many things we do not know'

42 Holgate et al. 2011

43 Good 2007, p. 117

44 Riadore 1843

45 WHO 1976; 2001; 2013.

46 Wakefield 2007

47 Reverso Context – omitting some misleading phrases – https://context.reverso.net/translation/

48 See Pullman 2002 on the connection between personal dignity and an aesthetics of wholeness, and for more on an aesthetic view of illness Kirmayer 2000; and also Radley 1999

49 Canguilhem 1991 p. 88

50 Ibid p. 184

51 See Harvey et al. 2012 for an account of how technologies such as genomics are creating personalised medicine

52 Peter Ellison quoted by Kleinman 1998

53 Final pathways conceal complex causes. A small range of physiological symptoms are the final pathway for the body's stress response, but they say nothing about the meaning or origin of the stress. Motor neurons are the final pathway for voluntary actions, but if you track the motor pathway backwards through the nervous system you will not arrive at 'the will'.

54 Conrad 2007 p. 4; p. 148

55 Illich 1976 p. 134

4

FEELINGS

FEELINGS

What kind of experience is illness? The last chapter defined illness as an essentially human phenomenon. A goldfish can have unpleasant feelings, but not those we call illness. When we describe a baby as ill, we are accepting her as a person rather some other kind of organism. Before we can understand much about how other individuals experience illness, we need to hear what they have to say, or if they cannot speak we must at least try to imagine what they would say if they could. We must be aware that we are only guessing; doctors who think they know what a patient feels because they know the medical diagnosis are conflating illness with disease.

Imagine Zola again. In Scene 1 she wakens in the night not feeling well. She says to herself that 'I am not quite myself'. All the physical and mental forms of illness we recognise are based on versions of this essentially human experience. Feeling 'not myself' would be a hopelessly vague piece of information from a diagnostic point of view, since there are probably as many ways of 'not being myself' as there are persons on the planet. But identifying the generic basis of illness experience makes it possible to respect the experiences associated with many different kinds of illness without needing to accommodate them to diagnostic categories such as 'psychosomatic', 'physical' and 'psychiatric'. Some of the fog that hangs over questions of diagnosis, classification, interpretation and treatment will be blown away if illness is primarily an existential state. The approach dissolves the contentious and troubling question of whether an illness is or is not 'real', leaving us with just two kinds: those that are real, and those that are feigned (I will leave the latter for the next chapter).

Becoming ill

What I am investigating here is the quality of being that becomes illness even though it could, in other circumstances, fit some alternative construct. I hope to get as close as possible to the first-person perspective of phenomenology. Phenomenology is not about what there is in the world, but about how the world is subjectively experienced. The philosopher Charles Sanders Peirce calls phenomenology the study of 'the collective total of all that is in any way or in any sense present to the mind, quite regardless of whether it corresponds to any real thing or not'.[1] This is difficult territory to explore without prejudicing descriptions of experience by framing them already as illness. Peirce says that we experience feelings before we can name them.

The two scenes I described in Chapter 1 identify distinct aspects of phenomenology. In Scene 2, Zola's feelings have resolved into the idea that she is ill, so that a narrative of illness can begin ('I went to the doctor who told me I had depression. Do you think I do? He wouldn't give me anything for it'). I regard this kind of phenomenology as secondary, to distinguish it from the primary phenomenology of Scene 1, where a person's experience has yet to be named or understood as something specific. In Scene 1 something has triggered feelings that might flow either towards a narrative of illness or else into an entirely different story (Perhaps she says to herself: 'My mother died a year ago, so of course I don't feel right' or 'my friend told me I'm always like this when my boys are away'). Primary phenomenology has nothing to do with disease. It exists as a question rather than a story, describing a liminal state in the territory between sickness and health. I call this transitional state of unwellness ill-being, in order to preserve some degree of ambiguity about its relationship to illness.

Published illness narratives begin after Scene 1, and they are less concerned with ill-being than with secondary phenomenology. In Havi Carel's book, which is grounded in the author's personal experience of a rare condition, the section on 'My Ill Body' records the experience of 'living in the shadow of chronic breathlessness'. The effects of breathlessness provide vital evidence about the experience of illness but so also would the quality of breathlessness, as a feeling (which Carel later explored more fully[2]). Arthur Kleinman's *Illness Narratives* is concerned with changed expectations and altered habits of body and mind that are the shadows cast by illness. I am equally interested in the sufferings that cast those shadows.[3]

Returning to Scene 1, Zola experiences the kind of unnameable disturbance that can 'break in upon us and destroy us'[4]: It is a 'showing', a phenomenon, that does not yet have a meaning. Peirce called this uninterpreted experience 'firstness'. Firstness is the pre-verbal splash of something that might (or might not) bring the language of illness in its wake. A person can feel 'wrong' without having any conception of what that wrongness signifies. Zola only begins to regard herself as ill when her experience has formed itself into signs that can be interpreted in that way. If she begins to see herself as ill in Scene 1, a more definite concept of illness will develop through dialogue, because her experience can then be 'read' by herself and others as a set of signs. A sign is something that stands for something for some person. From a semiotic point of view a symptom is a sign because by definition, it stands for some object that someone considers to exist.[5]

The concept of firstness trips you up when you try to write about it, because words are signs and firstness is by definition indescribable. Firstness does not come to you in Scene 1 already labelled as flu or epilepsy or even pain. You will only think of it in those ways if you are in a state of expectation, as Peirce calls it. The constructs I described in the previous chapter create just such a state of expectation, inviting someone like Zola to identify herself as ill. Perhaps what we experience in firstness is the closest we will get to knowing what it would be like to be a goldfish. We start with a somewhat fishlike awareness of difference, something we cannot think, let alone speak about. The feeling that I am not myself is a sign that points towards a cognitive object – the self – so it is not quite firstness, but it is the next best thing. Imagine seeing a friend's face and feeling a shock of difference, but nothing more. Only when you realise that he has shaved off his beard, say, or changed his glasses, or dyed his hair, do you have an object of consciousness that you can think and talk about: 'So that's what's happened!'

A state of expectation is often organised around a picture rather than a set of concepts. When a doctor hears a patient's symptoms, the diagnostic process often passes rapidly from what the patient says to a mental image of, say, a cancer, or a compressed nerve; or perhaps a physiological diagram of anaemia, or jaundice, or diabetes will be imagined. Zola's self-diagnosis might be at least as visual. In Scene 1 she could have a frightening image of ulceration or infection or death (it is the night!); or if she happens to be someone who expects divine punishment, perhaps she sees hell.

Our initial feelings of unwellness may seem indeterminate but there is intense social pressure to construct them as symptoms. Delayed diagnosis can be dangerous. 'If only you'd called me earlier', physicians used to say, as though a miraculous cure would have been possible if the patient had been quicker to recognise illness. Publicity campaigns constantly encourage us to recognise early signs of a heart attack (myocardial infarction) of stroke and of cancer.[6] The British Heart Foundation's website lists the early symptoms of myocardial infarction, positioning the reader as a candidate patient. It offers a phrase-book for the translation of raw experience into illness, so that the medical language game can begin when someone phones for help.

BOX 4.1: BRITISH HEART FOUNDATION ADVICE

The signs of a heart attack

Heart attack symptoms vary from one person to another. The most common signs of a heart attack are:

- chest pain: tightness, heaviness, pain or a burning feeling in your chest
- pain in arms, neck, jaw, back or stomach
- feeling light-headed
- become short of breath
- feeling nauseous or vomiting

Pain is a key symptom of myocardial infarction, as of many physical troubles, but it is a curious fact that pain is much easier to name than to describe. When a doctor and a patient talk about pain they both assume they 'know what they mean'. The questions doctors ask about pain are designed to classify the experience rather than to understand its quality. The doctor will listen for words like 'aching', 'stabbing' and 'sharp', and will be less interested in other words such as 'wrenching' and 'shattering' which happen to be less useful in the language game of diagnosis. The metaphors and similes we use when we describe pain to ourselves – 'tearing', 'scorching', 'stabbing', 'overwhelming' etc – express or create realities that may not correspond at all well to any concept of pain that doctors would recognise.

Pain is an elusive feeling. The International Association for the Study of Pain uses a definition of pain that barely describes it as an experience. Pain is simply 'unpleasant' - 'an unpleasant sensory and emotional experience associated with actual or potential tissue damage'.[10] This sounds like a concise combination of two essential criteria: (1) a specific experience and (2) a specific cause. But (2) turns out to be inessential according to the IASP: if a person describes a feeling in the language commonly used for pain caused by tissue damage, 'it should be accepted as pain'. As for (1), pain's specific quality, the IASP states that pain can be distinguished from other 'unpleasant abnormal experiences', asserting that these are not necessarily pain 'because, subjectively, they may not have the usual sensory qualities of pain'. But the IASP is silent on the question of what those 'usual sensory qualities' are. We are expected somehow to 'know what they mean'. The sufferer, not the IASP, must decide.

Another very common medical symptom is fatigue, which is if anything even less describable than pain. Fatigue can be 'overwhelming' and 'dreadful', but these words do not convey much. Research shows that descriptions of fatigue are vague and inconsistent.[7] People diagnosed with CFS/ME say that their fatigue has a special quality that is entirely different from everyday tiredness, and yet the words they use hardly help us know what they mean. We struggle to describe the phenomenology of fatigue itself, but does it have an 'itself'? What do people feel when fatigue 'breaks in'? Are feelings of fatigue mental or physical? The International Civil Aviation Organization defines fatigue by its practical effects[8] but at least one psychologist has despaired of characterising fatigue.[9]

Words such as pain and fatigue allow us to 'go on', as Wittgenstein puts it, with a medical language game.[11] A patient complained bitterly to me of what he called his pain, but rejected whatever suggestions or sympathy or support I offered. Everyone around him was frustrated until we helped him and his wife see that 'pain' was a loose and ineffective word for some other kind of experience. He had been caught up in a language game in which the word 'pain' was operating autonomously rather than being connected in a strong way with his phenomenal experience. He was using a natural-seeming concept, pain, as a 'floating signifier' that kept conversations going without anyone noticing its inadequacy. A diagnostic label often floats in this way. A medical conversation about 'my MS' or 'your CFS/ME' or 'his Alzheimer's' can go on indefinitely without ever connecting with anyone's lived reality. Illness is a floating signifier when the question of what it feels like is never asked.

Feeling ill

The jargon of medical symptoms is not how we describe feelings to each other. In place of the British Heart Foundation's formula, one writer describes his incipient heart attack as 'a dull, metallic pain in my chest and throat, and the taste of cement on my tongue'. Even the common cold defies description when 'you can't breathe, or think, or write or imagine what it was like before the onset of the cold'. Another writer uses a wonderful array of images for her CFS/ME: 'my head strangely fibrous, my body a wooden bulk I struggled to animate . . . An exhaustion thick as sod settled on my head and limbs'. In a semi-autobiographical novel, a woman's 'nervous prostration' (a medical phrase at the time) 'consists of every painful mental sensation, shame, fear, remorse, a blind oppressive confusion, utter weakness, a steady brain-ache that fills the conscious mind with crowding images of distress'. A story about HIV/AIDS has a man insisting that his skin lesions need 'more vivid language': they are 'good-sized blackcurrants on the surface of the skin'; his lungs feel like 'a pair of wrinkled socks'; he has 'the wrong kind of energy' and his body is fizzing 'like an electric razor that's been plugged into the wrong socket'.[12] These descriptions are creative, but not medical.

My patients often offered me evocative phrases to describe their experiences. Some belonged to recognizable idioms, such as 'rushing in the head', 'heavy legs' 'stuffing knocked out of me', or 'hollow inside' while others were utterly idiosyncratic. A woman told me that 'my leg is anxious'; I noted someone's description of 'a constant feeling of tension inside the body, indescribable, like strings pulling, sort of a pain'. Such phrases are useless from a diagnostic point of view, but they are often the best we can do in our efforts to communicate feelings. 'Let a sufferer try to describe a pain in his head to a doctor' writes Virginia Woolf,

> and language at once runs dry. There is nothing ready made for him. He is forced to coin words himself, and, taking his pain in one hand, and a lump of pure sound in the other (as perhaps the people of Babel did in the beginning), so to crush them together that a brand new word in the end drops out'.

We must use idiosyncratic language in illness because each of us is a pioneer when we are ill, walking across 'a virgin forest.... a snowfield where even the print of birds' feet is unknown'[13].

We can get a little closer to firstness through metaphors. The Czech poet Miroslav Holub says that talking about pain is like 'unpicking the stitch between blood and clay'.[14] When someone associates pain with a wrench or a needle or a sledge hammer we are getting the body's poetry rather than cognitive analysis. Quasi-metaphorical language sometimes shows something of what is happening to the body.[15] A person who feels metaphorically squashed perhaps is squashed in an almost physical sense; someone may shiver in a fever, but also with fear; a headache may have a splitting quality that seems also to pull both the body and the mind apart. People with CFS/ME who speak of heavy legs are trying to describe a bodily sensation and at the same time, perhaps, a less literal feeling of being weighed down. The Japanese language has a class of phrases called gitaigo mimetics that stand for feelings and also embody them. Siku siku means 'sobbing or in pain from a tooth or stomach ache'; biki biku is 'trembling, afraid or nervous, scared'; and muya muya means 'can't say what one wants to'.[16] A medical encounter often involves siku siku, biku biku, and especially muya muya. We are short of English equivalents. There is 'ouch!' as both a description and a demonstration of pain (a word may replace a cry, but the reverse is certainly true); we also have words like 'cringe', 'shudder', 'cower' and 'recoil', that can be either physical postures, or mimetics, or both at once, in much the way a person's symptoms can be directly and also metaphorically connected with the body. The language of feelings and of symptoms in English is limited, however, which is why John Koenig's online Dictionary of Obscure Sorrows is so appealing.[17]

Sufferers often trail off into a crude lament ('I'm feeling like shit!') that only says one thing: illness is bad. Symptoms may be difficult to describe but what we do know about them is that they are unwanted; we think of them as repellent in the aesthetic sense that I suggested in the last chapter (p. 27). My notes on someone diagnosed with chronic fatigue syndrome record what she told me: 'Feeling "not well". Wanting to be in bed. Not wanting to speak to people. Down. But: motivation still there? Annoyed. Sad. Feeling Awful'. Pain is awful. Nausea is also awful, and so are itches and many other symptoms of illness.[18]

When we say we feel ill, are we simply summarising the various kinds of badness that pain and fatigue and other unwanted feelings produce? I think not, because when bodily problems that count as illness turn up in everyday life we do not necessarily describe ourselves as ill. Pain is not exceptional for most people, and nor are fatigue, sleeplessness, dizziness, or itch. Another possibility is that illness is simply a word for feeling less comfortable than usual. I find this hard to accept since people who say they are ill usually look as though they are in the grip of something definite. The intense language people use when they complain of feeling 'awful', 'terrible' or 'ghastly' suggest something more than a random collection of discomforts.

Is badness all there is to illness? Rats know very well which stimuli are aversive and which are rewarding, and our primitive biological nature gives us the same information. We dislike nausea, itch, fatigue, pain and other illness symptoms in a rat-like way, but we cannot define illness simply as an unrewarding or unpleasing experience. Neither pain nor illness are mere subtractions from pleasure. They are burdens in themselves. We think of someone as coming 'down' with illness, and we make efforts to 'shake it off'. You only need to shake off something added, not something you lack. The language here is interesting. Perhaps the feeling of being burdened or overwhelmed makes illness feel phenomenologically like a thing, and maybe that is where the concrete grammar of illness and disease comes from. Illness is not just a burden, however, but also a restriction, making it something to wriggle out of as well as to shake off. It is a different way of being.

Ill-being

My subject here is the 'being' of illness. I call it ill-being rather than illness because it is not defined by physical or psychological criteria, and still less by medical diagnosis. Ill-being is unwellness, the sense that I am not myself. 'I am there, but not all there' says King George, echoing the poignant moment when another King, Lear, says 'My wits begin to turn'.[19] Physical afflictions have the same character as mental ones. Even in a bad cold we seem to lose the knack of being a normal self. Pain is experienced as illness only if it erodes one's normal sense of self. When Daudet writes that 'pain finds its way everywhere, into my vision, my feelings, my sense of judgement; it's an infiltration'[20] he is describing an ill-being that is rooted in the self.

Self

Whenever I feel that I am not myself, or when I imagine that illness is causing someone that I know well not to be himself, I am faced with a question I can otherwise ignore: what is a self? The concept of self is closely linked to the idea of an inner life, and for this reason has been vigorously attacked on theoretical grounds. Pierre Bourdieu berates 'the impostures of egoistic narcissism', insisting that there is 'externality at the heart of internality, banality in the illusion of rarity'.[21] One problem with this position is that it is impractical. We need a concept of self as a locus for attributes we all assume we have. In summarising the mind-body aporia, William James ends up close to the concept of a soul; Anatole Broyard unashamedly calls the soul 'the part of you that you summon up in emergencies'.[22] Illness is an emergency that cannot afford to be philosophically fastidious.

I am arguing for the self or soul, not as a metaphysical truth but as a way of conceptualizing empirical realities. The uniqueness of ill-being is a fact, not an illusion created by an individual's particular perceptions and beliefs about the self. In illness the 'other life' that Canguilhem describes[23] must be lived by a body that from an empirical standpoint is more or less unique, and experienced from a singular position in the world. It is a fact that the person who dies will be me, and me alone, just as your pain belongs entirely to your self. An illness narrative is the story of a single, unique life. Decentring the self, as in Buddhism, does not alter this truth. The Buddha is quoted as saying that 'you yourselves must strive; the Buddhas only point the way'.[24] Medical discourse tries to sweep the 'I' into a 'psychosocial' domain, but in the Sahara Desert you may not know whether you are in Algeria or Libya, and when you are in the terrain of illness you will not make rigid distinctions between physical, mental and social distress.[25] Together, they form the field of a body-self's experience.

I think of the self as discovered, or perhaps created, in relationships, primarily between an infant and a parent.[26] We imagine the self's attributes as (1) uniqueness; (2) integrity (oneness); (3) temporal continuity; (4) free will; and (5) moral responsibility. Illness threatens each of these at times.

Uniqueness

The sense of being a unique human being is undermined when one is categorized as typical of some diagnosis and it is hard to hold on to while being rolled into a scanner or swabbed for surgery.

Integrity

The words health and healing come to us from an old English term for wholeness and the advice we often give ourselves in the confused firstness of ill-being is 'Pull yourself together!' Psychiatry is much concerned with splits in the self but the body-self's sense of integrity is also threatened in physical illness, for example by an enhanced awareness of the body or by feeling separated from an injured body part. Daudet feels himself being infiltrated by pain; Siri Hustvedt senses the presence within her of 'an uncontrollable other'.[27]

Continuity

Chronic illness almost inevitably interrupts the self's continuity of being, as though one version is being replaced by another.

Will and responsibility

Illness is a threat to autonomy and excuses a sick person in some degree from moral responsibilities.

Qualities of ill-being

Illness is a shrunken way of being.[28] The complaint that I am not myself implies that I am less myself. In ecstasy, which means 'standing outside', you embrace a larger world and may think you are more yourself. In illness you are forced to stand inside your shrivelled self; it is an 'enstasy'. This is obvious in the illness we call depression, and also in anxiety, where feelings are so monotonously self-referential. The same thinning out of the self occurs in physical illness, where it may be shrunk to 'a fiery motionless particle' whose sole remaining aim is 'to resist destruction, to survive and to be in its own madness of being. In illness one can 'wake up in the night, with nothing beyond a mere sense of existing. But the place, the time, the personal sense of self, are completely lost. Not a single idea'; one can find oneself 'clinging to that old self that is fast floating away'.[29]

Illness feels worse when you are away from home. 'A terrible feeling swept over me, a dread felt as a stomach punch. It was too late, I was very ill and I was in New York, three thousand miles from home, in a strange hotel'.[30] Illness is a strange hotel in which the environment feels as wrong as you do yourself. This is partly because the world no longer delivers its normal possibilities. In prolonged seasickness, as William James says, 'every good, terrestrial or celestial, is imagined only to be turned from with disgust'. All kinds of appetite are reduced in any kind of physical and mental ill-being. The world is a stranger to you. Perhaps you feel, as Anatole Broyard does, something equivalent to the anthropological concept of 'soul loss': 'a sense of terrible emptiness, a feeling that your soul has abandoned your ailing body like rats deserting a sinking ship. When your soul leaves, the illness rushes in'.[31]

At the same time, you are a stranger to your body, or rather, the body forces itself into consciousness in a disturbing way. In illness we become acutely aware that 'we live not alone, but chained to a creature of a different kingdom, whole worlds apart, who has no knowledge of us and by whom it is impossible to make ourselves understood: our body . . . '. Despite being enjoined to 'listen to the body', what we hear makes no sense. Nor will the sick body listen to us. '[T]o ask pity of our body is like discoursing in front of an octopus, for which our words can have no more meaning than the sound of the tides, and with which we should be appalled to find ourselves condemned to live'.[32] Svenaeus contrasts such feelings with the 'homelike being-in-the-world' of health, in which the body can access the environment transparently. He uses the word 'unhomelikeness'[33], echoing the German word umheimlich, which means unhomelike and also uncanny. According to Freud, something is uncanny when it is familiar and at the same time unfamiliar[34], and the body sometimes has this quality in illness. A feeling of unreality, remoteness or uncanniness can afflict the sick person if the body's normally taken-for-granted insides are producing strange sensations. The innards were a field for divine action and then for philosophical speculation for the ancient Greeks[35]; medical knowledge has made the body more familiar to us from a technical point of view, but the internal source of symptoms is not experienced as a physiological diagram but as something strange and unfamiliar. The body becomes an alien presence when the lungs feel like wrinkled socks or the tongue tastes of cement.

The enstasy of ill-being separates the well from the sick. There is something uncanny about being with a person you know well who is delirious, or whose face is swollen beyond recognition. Another person's pain can have the same distancing effect because, as Elaine Scarry writes, it has 'the remote character of some deep subterranean fact, belonging to an invisible geography'[36]. The transformation of the self, the body and relationships is only to be expected because ill-being is 'another life'.

Awareness of one's smallness and helplessness generates a sense of dread: 'I am sick, I must die. Lord, have mercy on us!'; 'What have I done, and what do I fear?'.[37] In acute illness someone finds herself 'on a narrow ledge over a pit that she knew to be bottomless, though she could not comprehend it; the ledge was her childhood dream of danger, and she strained back against a reassuring wall of granite at her shoulders, staring into the pit . . . '.[38] The ontological insecurity that RD Laing describes in a psychiatric context is experienced in physical illness as well. It is a state in which you feel 'in a literal sense, more dead than alive'. You lose your sense of continuity and coherence, and you are liable to feel 'more insubstantial than substantial, and unable to assume that the stuff [you are] made of is genuine, good, valuable'.[39] All forms of ill-being have these effects in one degree or another. Even a common cold can make me feel less 'substantial' and less 'genuine, good, valuable', and nausea makes it impossible to carry on as the self I normally am, or even to be sure that such a self still exists.

In medical terminology a symptom that is decisively diagnostic of something is pathognomonic. The features of ill-being I have been identifying are not pathognomonic of any physical or mental condition. They are not even pathognomonic of illness. They reflect a transformation of the body-self that is also experienced in other, very different contexts. Chitra Ramaswamy's account of pregnancy could almost be a description of illness: 'My body remained a stranger. I didn't feel pregnant, but I did feel altered, like a walking phantom limb. No, even more transported'. In describing her sickness, she uses words with poetic distinctiveness, just as ill people do ('A peculiar taste in the mouth, smooth and slightly metallic like a conker pressed to the tongue. It was a shimmering nausea, heated, rich and thirst-inducing . . . '); and she points out how the problem of the self 'doubles, trebles, multiplies when there are at least two people inside one body'.[40] Pregnancy is not an illness, but it evidently can feel like one. Nor is disability an illness, as I said earlier, but I often watched physically injured people move, over a period of weeks or months or years, from a state of distressed helplessness to one in which the same impairments had become a more or less neutral fact about their lives. It was as though they had been ill and had become well. A person would sometimes sink back towards ill-being for a while, even though the level of physical impairment had not changed much.

I am using the word ill-being to describe a crisis of the body-self that can arise before the question of illness has been settled. Ill-being is made of essentially the same material as other forms of existential distress. If I feel that I am not myself, if I have a sense of shrinkage, if my body and surroundings seem unhomelike and unappetizing, I may use medical language but there are also alternative genres of the troubled self.[41]

The body is just as central to philosophical and spiritual versions of the troubled self as it is to illness narratives. Sartre's character Roquentin, for example, in La Nausée, writes that 'I have a broken spring: I can move my eyes but not my head. The head is all pliable and elastic, as though it had been simply set on my neck; if I turn it, it will fall off'. The same physicality runs through Georges Bernanos' commentary on boredom. It is a sort of dust that you breathe and eat; you must be constantly on the go to shake this 'drizzle of ashes' off your face and hands. John Bunyan's spiritual and physical restlessness is similar: 'Thus did I wind, and twine, and shrink, under the burden that was upon me; which burden also did so oppress me that I could neither stand, nor go, nor lie, either at rest or quiet'.[42] The psalms, which inspired Bunyan's language, abound with expressions of embodied distress. In Psalm 102, for example, 'My heart is struck down like grass and has withered; I forget to eat my bread. Because of my loud groaning my bones cling to my flesh' and in Psalm 38 'my loins are filled with burning, and there is no soundness in my flesh. I am utterly spent and crushed; I groan because of the tumult of my heart'.[43]

When the self 'speaks' it does so through what it knows – the body. I do not think there is a different, exclusively spiritual register in which our experience as selves can be expressed.[44] The feeling that John Berryman describes 'here near the bottom of my chest, a loop of cold, on the right'[45] is not the poetic equivalent of some alternative, non-bodily experience; it implies neither a medical diagnosis nor its opposite. We experience ill-being through the body and soul together. As Fernando Pessoa writes:

> There are some deep-seated griefs so subtle and pervasive that it is difficult to grasp whether they belong to our soul or to our body, whether they come from a malaise brought on by pondering on the futility of life, or whether they are caused rather by an indisposition in some chasm within ourselves – the stomach, liver or brain.[46]

What is illness?

In this exploration of feelings, I began by trying to get as close as possible to firstness. By its nature firstness is indescribable because it is a primal experience that is not yet 'about' anything. However, I tried to pare down the 'aboutness' (intentionality) of feelings of illness to the point where experience is less a question of causes, effects and meanings than of raw, uninterpreted phenomena.[47] From there I investigated the quality of feelings that sometimes are and sometimes are not called symptoms. My objective was to define an experience I call ill-being in order not to commit it, in advance, to the construct of illness. Ill-being is an existential state, not a diagnosis. I am not using the concept of ill-being as a synonym for illness. Ill-being can be the core experience of someone with a medically validated illness, but also of someone whose claim to be ill has been rejected, and a person with no interest in a medical description could have similar experiences. Ill-being is a particular version of experiences that are common to 'trouble, sorrow, need . . . and other adversity'. I ended the last chapter with the suggestion that illness is medically-defined suffering. Naming ill-being as illness defines need in such a way as to draw the person towards medical sources of help.

By viewing illness as a species of personal being we can attend to a person's subjective realities without needing to label them as 'physical', 'psychosomatic', or 'mental'. Such labels imply mechanisms that are important in other contexts, but they do not determine an individual's experience. Many different kinds of illness are experientially equivalent. A group of Canadian psychiatrists resist this conclusion, stating that mental illnesses are unlike other illnesses because they affect 'the very core of one's being through a range of experiences and phenomena of varying severity that alter the individual's thinking, perception and consciousness about the self, others and the world'.[48] I disagree. The self's dislocation is especially severe in psychiatric conditions such as psychosis, but the core of one's being can be profoundly disrupted also by physical symptoms.

An important implication of the approach I have taken is that the grounds for assessing the 'realness' of illness are entirely subjective. Someone who sincerely claims to be ill is ill, just as someone who reports pain is in pain.

Notes

1 Peirce 1931–1966 Vol 1 para 284
2 Macnaughton & Carel 2016; Carel 2018
3 Breathlessness: Carel 2013 p. 35; Macnaughton & Carel 2016; Carel 2018. narrative: Harvey & Koteyko 2013 (Chapter 3); Kleinman 1988
4 Heidegger 1962 p. 193
5 In the jargon of modern medicine, a symptom is something the patient complains of and a sign is an objective manifestation of disease, but from a semiotic point of view these are two species of signifier. For Peirce's definition see Merrell 2001 and Peirce 1931–66 Vol 2 para 228. A sign can convey meaning unconsciously. Jakob von Uexküll (1934/ 2010) argues that rats and birds and even tics respond to signs. Each of these, like ourselves, has what Uexküll calls an Umwelt within which certain signs have significance in terms of an organism's practical life.
6 On cancer information, see www.cancerresearchuk.org/about-cancer/; on heart attack, see British Heart Foundation website, www.bhf.org.uk/informationsupport/conditions/ heart-attack
7 See Standen et. al. 2015
8 ICAO 2012
9 Muscio (1921) said that 'the term should be absolutely banished from scientific discussion'
10 Williams & Craig 2016
11 Wittgenstein 1967; language game 244–246; pain 151–155
12 Heart attack: Mehmedinović 2012; common cold: Diamond 1998 p. 7; CFS/ME: Wall 2005; nervous prostration: Gilman 1892; HIV/AIDS: Mars-Jones E. 'Slim'. In: Mars-Jones 1987
13 Woolf 1926
14 Brief Reflection on the Word Pain (Holub 2006)
15 When Hamlet asks: 'What should such fellows as I do crawling between earth and heaven?', crawling is metaphorical, but also almost literal – an example for the critic IA Richards
16 Occhi 1999
17 See www.dictionaryofobscuresorrows.com/. For example: 'rubatosis n. the unsettling awareness of your own heartbeat, whose tenuous muscular throbbing feels less like a metronome than a nervous ditty'
18 Philosophers and theologians are too preoccupied with pain as the paradigm for suffering. They would do well to think more about other less heroic-sounding symptoms. There is nothing remotely noble about vomiting
19 Alan Bennett. *The Madness of King George*; Shakespeare, *King Lear*, Act 3 scene 2
20 Daudet 2002 p. 23
21 Bourdieu 1990 p. 21
22 Broyard 1992, p. 40. To get behind contemporary anxieties about the self, see William James' *Principles of Psychology* Volume 1 Chapter 10 The consciousness of Self, Chapter 8 The Mind-stuff theory.
23 Canguilhem 1991 – see Chapter 4
24 Buddharakkhita 1996. Chapter 20, Maggavagga: The Path, verse 276.

25 'The map is not the territory' – Korzybski 1994 Chapter 4.
26 'When I look I am seen, so I exist. I can now afford to look and see. I now look crea-tively and what I apperceive I also perceive; in fact I take care not to see what is not there to be seen'. Winnicott 2005 p. 154
27 Hustvedt 2011, p. 47
28 See Ayo and Ayo 2008, p.115
29 'Motionless particle.' Porter 1939/1965; 'wake up in the night' Daudet 2002 p. 43; 'clinging to that old self' Wall 2005 p. 13
30 Wall 2005 p. 6
31 Broyard 1992, p. 40
32 Proust 1920/1982, Part I Chapter 1, p. 308
33 Svenaeus 2011
34 Freud 1919/2003
35 Holmes 2010
36 Scarry 1985, p.4
37 'I am sick.': Thomas Nashe Litany in a Time of Plague, 1600; 'What have I done': Robert Louis Stevenson. The Sick Child 1887
38 Porter 1939/1965
39 Laing 1960 p. 42
40 Ramaswamy 2016; see also Gavin Francis' (2018) essays on pregnancy, puberty and other bodily transformations
41 Recalling Bakhtin's concept of speech genres – see previous chapter
42 Sartre 1938; Bernanos 1937; Bunyan J. Grace Abounding to the Chief of Sinners. 1666, para 165
43 Psalm 102:3–5 and 38:7–8. English Standard Version (Anglicised). See also Shabbat Shalom Magazine 3/11/2015 for examples of how embodiment is imagined in Hebrew scripture: 'Guts, *rechem*, have compassion (Gen 43:30); kidneys, *kilyot*, convey instruction (Ps 16:7); the heart, *leb*, thinks (Ezek 38:10), feels (Ps 39:4) or understands (1 Kgs 3:9); the ears, *ozenim*, understand (Prov 18:15). The flesh, *basar*, is troubled (Jer 12:12), knows (Ezek 21:10), is spiritual (Joel 3:1), worships (Isa 66:23; Ps 145:21) . . . Man may think with his body and eat with his soul, just as he may think with his soul and eat with his body . . . *nephesh* (soul) and *basar* (flesh) are often interchangeable (Num 31:35; cf. Ps 145:21). Shabbat Shalom Magazine 3/11/2015 The Hebrew Concept of Helth https://bit.ly/323jDMR
44 Cromby 2015
45 Dreamsong 207. Berryman 1969
46 Pessoa 1991. Quoted by kind permission of Serpent's Tail
47 A thought or sign has intentionality if it is connected with or 'about' something in the world
48 Malla et al. 2015. The divergence between my position and these authors narrows or disappears when the distinction between illness and disease is taken into account

5

APPEARANCES

The previous chapter tracked an episode of unwellness from its firstness, and this one continues along the same path, from the point where a person's feelings appear in the world under the banner of illness. A sufferer must in some way make illness apparent before there is any possibility of help. Whether illness is framed as physical, as 'mental' or as something between the two, doctors and others will judge whether people are 'really' ill from the way they look and sound and behave. Viewing illness from the outside requires us to follow the contours that the social constructs of illness, disease and medicine carve out for us, and from now on I will be using the words 'illness' and 'illnesses', because these are the concepts that anyone complaining of feeling ill must use in order to be understood in the social world. Ill-being, as an experience and as a source of need, must be constantly borne in mind, however. Personal feelings are easily overshadowed by the construct of illness.

Think of the many settings in which illness offers itself as a possible reality. Sometimes the idea of illness is so obvious that the individual can hardly escape the glare of other people's concern. At such moments the sick body seems to say it all. Ill-being sometimes expresses itself as a lament that does not necessarily ask for anything: 'I am sick, I must die!'. Often, however, feelings of illness are expressed in an acute sense of need ("Help me mummy!") or as a gesture of incapacity ('I think I'll go home, I'm sickening for something'; 'please finish this job – I'm not well'). These are human encounters in which some other person functions as an observer of the body. Just as a doctor looks for physical signs of disease, so you may stand over your sleeping child wondering if she is sick; or you might keep an eye on a colleague at work, noticing that he is 'not himself'.

The question of how the experience of illness is made visible concerns both the sufferer and others. The ill person might ask: 'Am I unwell enough to be counted as ill?'; if so: 'How do I communicate my needs?'. There is the ever-present danger that symptoms will be dismissed as trivial, unexceptional, or even unreal. Meanwhile, those who encounter the ill person have similar questions in mind. They are making assessments based on what an ill person ought to look like, and on who deserves to be cared for.

I will begin by outlining two ways in which an ill person is commonly seen, firstly as an object of biological diagnosis (does the body look abnormal in a medical sense? is it sick?) and secondly as an object of behavioural diagnosis (is he acting like someone who is 'really ill'?). The chapter then develops an account of how the body makes feelings of illness apparent.

The diagnostic gaze

Many people examine an ill person with a diagnostic eye. A parent classifies a child as ill enough not to go to school; an employer estimates someone's ability to carry on working; a worried friend sizes you up: 'Are you ill, or just unhappy?' A doctor looks at a patient, deciding what action is needed. Appearances matter in all these situations because they so powerfully influence human responses. A picture captivates us. An image of sincerity creates one way of seeing and knowing what a person does, but a suspicion of 'abnormal illness behaviour' creates another. Once we get the idea of disease, the pictures that occur to us tend to close off the possibility that a person is not unwell, and conversely the needs of someone who looks 'a picture of health' are often underestimated. Even the most technical of diagnoses flows in some degree from a person's appearance, and the same is true of the informal diagnoses people give each other.

Biological diagnosis

What we often see when we look at an ill person is a sick body. The primary purpose of physical inspection is to yield a diagnosis. To name an illness is sometimes to name its treatment: something that looks like a snake bite calls for antivenom, just as the appearance of infection calls for antibiotics. A medical plan of action can often be mapped out at a glance. In my experience even a momentous diagnosis such as motor neurone disease could frequently be made on the basis of a very few symptoms and two or three physical signs. The power of the medical gaze is so obvious at such times that doctors are liable to attend more to the body than to feelings. I was not the top-hatted power-monger of sociological myth, but my usefulness as a doctor sometimes depended primarily on a very restricted medical gaze.

In Chapter 3 I showed that any diagnosis, valid or otherwise, can create realities rather than merely documenting them (p. 19). A diagnosis, even one made informally at home, transforms the person into someone 'with' an illness, so that from then on everything the body is and does takes on an aura of sickness. Rather than revealing precisely what a person is complaining of, a diagnosis such as 'flu' or 'cancer' suggests how the person ought to appear, how they should behave, and to some extent also how they 'must' feel. No need for a patient to describe feelings if the symptoms of X or Y or Z are matters of public record. Deviations from the standard picture are swept aside if they do not fit with what the diagnosis requires.

Behavioural diagnosis

The sociologist David Mechanic defined illness behaviour as 'the ways in which given symptoms may be differentially perceived, evaluated and acted (or not acted) upon by different kinds of persons'.[1] Mechanic's ambition was to identify groups of persons in much the way that medical classification does. As with medical diagnosis, the study of illness behaviour implies the possibility of defining social norms, hence the psycho-sociological diagnosis of 'abnormal illness behaviour'. Classifying a person's behaviour has implications similar to those of biological diagnosis. Everything the ill person says or does comes to be seen in a particular light. Behavioural diagnosis also in a sense creates realities, just as a biological label does, because it has the same tendency to regard whatever it sees as typical of a 'diagnostic picture'. For example, a person's 'fatigue' would be deemed typical of CFS/ME in medical terms, but through a sociological lens inactivity might be diagnosed as a facet of illness behaviour. Feelings are as peripheral to the goals of behavioural diagnosis as they are to those of medicine, since both perspectives aim to explain an individual's situation in terms of extrapersonal mechanisms.

Social and cultural factors profoundly influence the way people react to feelings of unwellness. Where one person reaches for the paracetamol and seeks medical advice, another is more reluctant to use the idea of illness as a description of distress. Patterns of illness-related behaviour reflect the environments in which they are learned, so that the appearances of illness vary between social groups, and between families. The most thoroughly social aspect of illness behaviour concerns the management of identity. Illness involves looking like someone who is sick and abandoning the appearances of health. These are processes that the sociologist Irving Goffman calls impression management, although illness is not among the examples he primarily uses in his book *The Presentation of Self in Everyday Life*.[2] Management of identity is a special challenge in chronic illness, as discussed in Chapter 8 (pp. 94–95), but the elements of impression management are present even in the most trivial of illnesses. At work, for example, we use our ills as excuses and justifications for what we have done, and as disclaimers that ask people to make less demands on us because we are not feeling well ('don't expect much from me today, I'm not feeling too good').[3]

What people see are signs. Stigma, which etymologically simply means 'sign', stands for social forces that have profound effects on identity. Stigma is either directly visible as scars and deformities or else comes to us as mental images such as of madness or contamination. Either way it creates pictures that are very liable to hold us all captive. Stigma's power to over-ride rational human relationships is extraordinary.[4] In one experiment, pedestrians waiting at a road crossing stood measurably further away from a researcher with a facial mark on her face than they did when the same person had no blemish.[5] This was compelling evidence that most of us tend to be repelled by even minor abnormalities of the body. We use stigma to classify people in the same way that doctors use symptoms and biological abnormalities as diagnostic criteria. The overlap between illness and badness that I described in Chapter 3 (p. 36) helps to explain why deformities and other deviations from the norm are so often shunned. Stigma separates the beautiful from the ugly, the good from the bad, the normal from the abnormal. These dichotomies might track back to a primal effort, described by the anthropologist Mary Douglas, to keep oneself spiritually as well as physically pure.[6] Hence the connotations of stigma are liable to spread like an oil slick, to the point that an ill person can seem to be morally culpable. Fear of contagion, borrowed from the stigma of infectious disease, is sometimes a background worry. I have occasionally been asked if MS can be caught (which it cannot).

The dynamics of stigma have the same social sources in mental as in physical illness. Psychiatric illnesses are liable to evoke fear, or even an atavistic sense of disgust. An ill-defined and invisible illness such as CFS/ME makes people uneasy. A young man with this diagnosis described how he was 'embarrassed of falling behind . . . resentful of [friends] for not calling and embarrassed of my "prolonged childhood" . . . One so-called friend called me a "loser", the other a "malingerer." They thought that it was all in my head'.[7]

Seeing through the patient

'One recalls with great shame the epilepsy scandal of 1940, when many experienced neurologists were tricked by mother's darlings who wished to avoid military service',[8] said a London surgeon called Mr A Dickson Wright, in his presidential address to the Hunterian Society in 1955. His title was 'How Patients have Deceived me'. Dickson Wright was pouring scorn on young men he considered to be malingering, i.e. manufacturing symptoms for the sake of personal advantage. His lecture attracted an exceptionally large audience of doctors and the vote of thanks suggests that they were vastly entertained. Doctors love to tell each other stories of times when they have caught out malingerers. Most of the neurologists who trained me took pride in their ability to 'see through' patients who did not have organic (i.e. 'genuine') neurological disorders. They shared Dickson Wright's simplistic (and decidedly masculine) ethos. There was a clear distinction to be made between two species of medical symptoms, the real and the fake. Fake illnesses reduced wartime fighting capacity. They were also an economic threat in peacetime, producing bogus claims for benefits and insurance payouts.

'Seeing through' is a form of behavioural diagnosis, but with a perspective that is personal and moral rather than social. It regards the person as a protagonist to be resisted rather than understood. The glee with which I have seen neurologists catch their patients out has an edge of anger in it: 'You are trying to fool me but I'm too clever for you!'. There is perhaps a touch of envy in the way one British neurologist describes how Weir Mitchell, a celebrated 19th century American neurologist, was able to 'prevent what we now call illness behaviour' (note:

illness behaviour, which among physicians is often taken to be a synonym for abnormal illness behaviour); he writes that Mitchell, 'attending a lady, sick unto death . . . dismissed his assistants from the room, then soon left himself. Asked of her chances of survival he remarked: 'Yes, she will run out of the door in two minutes; I set her sheets on fire. A case of hysteria'.[9] What matters diagnostically in these scenarios is to exclude fakeness from medical attention rather than to view it as a human problem in its own right. The diagnostic gaze sees nothing more once it has penetrated the person's sham symptoms.

Doctors who think they 'see through' their patients rarely pause to consider any motivation that is more complicated than simple fraud. The result is that the field of illness mimicry is in a considerable muddle, because there are many reasons why people without credible symptoms produce the appearance of illness. Malingering is forgery, aspiring to a perfect replica of some medical picture, usually for purposes of gain.[10] Munchausen's syndrome, as Richard Asher called it[11], is more complicated because its motivations are obscure. Still more puzzling is Munchausen's-by-proxy, the now outmoded label for the manufacturing of symptoms in a child or other susceptible person rather than in oneself. Dickson Wright's lecture described more cases of these latter kinds than malingerers. Several had undergone painful medical procedures (one had three amputations) without any obvious gain. Here are some examples from my own experience:

> *Gordon was brought to the eye department saying that he had suddenly been struck blind in both eyes. There aren't many causes of sudden, total loss of sight, so the oph-thalmologists were intrigued. After running innumerable investigations, they despaired of finding the cause and referred him to the social worker to be registered as blind, only to discover that he was already on the blind register. For some reason this man was re-enacting efforts to seek medical attention for a problem he had probably had for years.*
>
> *I was alerted to Willie when I was working in the far north of Scotland. Just as I was putting up an intravenous infusion for him, a GP phoned to inform me that this man had visited many medical centres to the south of us, always seeking help for his non-existent diabetes and his non-existent epilepsy. When he was rumbled, he disappeared without a word.*
>
> *John, a young man with severe, neurologically proven epilepsy was also subject to convulsive movements and blackouts that could be shown to be 'non-epileptic'. I had a quiet talk with him during one of his frequent hospital admissions, and informed him that we knew from EEG recordings that not all his funny turns were epilepsy. I remember him suggesting rather sheepishly that 'perhaps I do it for attention'.*
>
> *Elaine presented with a history of sudden blindness in one eye. We used a red filter in front of her good eye to show that she could read words in tiny red lettering with her supposedly sightless eye. She had a scar across her forehead following a neurosurgical operation performed the last time she had presented to a hospital with blindness.*

Willie had no prospect of gaining from his feigned symptoms. He was exposing himself again and again to the experience of being found out. His rapid movement through Scotland might have been a flight from exposure, or was he racing towards his next humiliation? Much the same could be said of Gordon's blindness. John, on the other hand, seemed to be as confused as we were by his symptoms, which were as much a burden for him as his epilepsy. Elaine was not fraudulent. Even when we demonstrated that she could see, she was trembling with obvious emotion, saying 'It's the darkness that frightens me'.

Deliberate mimicry of illness must not be confused with unconsciously producing the appearance of disease. In neurology we used to call this hysteria, an obsolete term for which there is no satisfactory alternative.[12]

> *Wahid had been diagnosed with multiple sclerosis. He was paraplegic (both legs paralysed) and incontinent, and he had all the appearances of someone with irreparable damage to the spinal cord. Wahid suffered frequent crises and was often admitted to the hospital where I was working as a junior doctor. Late one evening I went wearily to the front of the hospital to receive Wahid yet again from the emergency ambulance, expecting him to be on a stretcher as usual. He sprang out of the ambulance, abandoning his wheelchair and twirling his crutches in the air. During a long wait for the ambulance his GP had hypnotised him, with dramatic effect.*

Wahid's transformation proved that his symptoms and disabilities did not have a straightforward neurological explanation, since spinal cord damage cannot be cured by hypnosis. Whether he was conscious or unconscious of manufacturing symptoms was uncertain. At any rate, he voluntarily surrendered equipment supplied to people with paraplegia, and sacrificed any benefits there might have been from the medical attention he had been receiving before he was cured. He abandoned the appearance of MS.

> *When she was four, Rowena suddenly developed a limp. She was about to leave her home for the first time, to be looked after by grandparents during a house move. The limp recovered rapidly with reassurance.*

Little Rowena did have something to gain from her lameness, since her mum might pay more attention to her if she was ill or, better still, keep her at home rather than letting her go to her grandparents, but she was not conscious of playing a game.

Whether one adopts a Freudian perspective or not there is no denying the connection between unconscious processes and bodily function. The brain does not just think and feel. It also has a role in the immune system and in respiration, digestion, and every aspect of bodily function. There is a continuum between physical changes that routinely inform us about subliminal or unconscious feelings (blushing, nervousness, sexual arousal, etc) and those that more closely resemble medical symptoms (palpitations, diarrhoea or headaches, for example). The construct of illness hovers over these phenomena because they can be framed either as the psychosomatics of everyday life or else as pathological disorders. For them to be seen as illness the patient must show and describe them in the right way. People diagnosed with CFS/ME strive to assert their identities as sick persons partly because they know that there are people who think they can 'see through' their troubles and who want to rob them of the right to appear ill.

The performance of illness

A malingerer who wishes to be viewed as ill must display the right kind of body but also the right kinds of behaviour. The same is true of anyone who wants feelings to be regarded as feeling ill. 'Once someone has chosen to fall ill' writes Jonathan Miller, 'he has to apply for the role of patient: he auditions for the part by reciting his complaint as vividly and as convincingly as he can'.[13] Illness must be performed in accordance with the cultural expectations of both medical and non-medical audiences. Family members, doctors, employers and others look for non-verbal as well as verbal evidence of illness. Anatole Broyard points up the paradox of illness performance: 'There is an etiquette to being sick. I never act sick with my doctor'.[14]

How to malinger

People who manufacture symptoms and disabilities are generally hoping for some practical advantage such as a day off work, discharge from military service or financial compensation. The best ways to convince others that you are ill will vary according to your audience. Styles of malingering will be different in other cultures, and I can only speak from my own Anglo-American perspective.[15] If you are a child not wanting to go to school you may only need to convince your mum that you are ill. Saying 'I feel awful' just might be sufficient. In a doctor's consulting room, however, it is not enough just to say you feel unwell. You must be prepared to answer the doctor's questions, reporting your complaints in terms that can be translated by the doctor into symptoms – symptoms of some recognizable illness. Piling on too many symptoms reduces your chance of being believed.[16]

To be credible the malingerer must show as well as tell. If you say you feel awful then you must also look awful, and everyone needs to see that you are as ill as you claim to be. You cannot look full of beans and expect anyone to believe that you are depressed, or look entirely relaxed when describing severe anxiety, even though people who are depressed or anxious often do mask their problems. If you complain to the doctor of excruciating pain you cannot sit motionless for ten minutes, even though there are stoical people who can do that. Appropriate 'pain behaviour' such as wincing and fidgeting and groaning and changing bodily position is advisable.

Histrionic and extreme behaviour will undermine your credibility. Good liars, like good actors, know the appearance of emotions such as remorse, sympathy and indignation. Successful malingerers are aware of the ways in which people with genuine distress usually behave, just as they know what patterns of symptoms and signs are most credible from a medical point of view.

How to be ill

If you really are ill you must follow the malingerers' guidelines. The need to communicate symptoms credibly – to perform them – is just as great in genuine as in manufactured illness. Making one's symptoms understandable to other people is not a straightforward task. There is a great risk of being disbelieved or misunderstood if you lack the communicative skills and cultural sensitivities that a successful malingerer has. For a doctor to see what is wrong it is best to produce just the right number of complaints, in just the right order, along with just the right amount of illness behaviour. When the surgeon places a hand on the skin overlying an inflamed appendix the patient will be well advised not to suppress the pain that the examination produces, but nor should he over-react. The patient's performative task is to behave in a way that fits with what he is feeling and that also matches the conventional appearances of those feelings. Admittedly, there is hardly a need to act out the symptoms of acute appendicitis or malaria since their bodily effects are obvious, but the outcomes of those situations hinge on the diagnosis of disease. Communicating one's feelings of illness is a separate, more challenging task.

Individuals vary greatly in their ability to match what they look like with what they inwardly feel, which is why some sick people find it hard to perform illness in a credible way. I once asked a man complaining of walking difficulty to demonstrate his problem and his wife protested 'Come on Albert, you can walk worse than that!'. Albert, probably dragged to the doctor under protest, was determined to minimise his symptoms rather than admit to his very real difficulties. Some people are so stoical that the doctor does not notice that there is anything wrong. At the other extreme are those whose dramatic symptoms and behaviour suggest a strenuous effort to be believed. Lack of confidence that one's feelings will be given credence can lead to exaggerated versions of underlying symptoms. Some people shower the doctor with so many complaints that whatever difficulties they have are virtually uninterpretable. The bizarre, inconsistent symptoms and incongruous behaviour of some of my patients made it impossible to know what, if anything, was wrong. Colleagues might diagnose them with borderline personality disorder, but this label was not in itself a guide to their feelings. I thought of such patients as lacking the ability to communicate whether they were ill or not. They could not see themselves as others saw them; they probably could hardly see themselves at all. I often wondered whether they grew weary of their illness performances and were like the Munchhausen patients I described earlier, and might have had an unconscious desire to be rejected by the doctor.

Sam was a young man who was unable to walk. He had joined a programme of rehabilitation that involved counselling sessions during which he disclosed to us a history of sexual trauma and domestic abuse. There was no evidence that his impairments had a neurological basis and we felt sure they were related to psychological stress. Whilst being brought to a day centre in a minibus he noticed that one of the tyres of his wheelchair was deflated, came out of the chair, pumped up the tyre, and then resumed his posture as a wheelchair-bound person.

> *Susie came to see the neurologist with her husband. She was complaining of severe walking difficulties. The examining neurologist asked her to walk a few yards to assess the problem, and then respectfully requested her to demonstrate how she used to walk when she was well – upon which she walked normally across the room.*

The key to these puzzling scenarios lies in the borderland between reality and make-believe. Children can switch rapidly between different realities, performing a self-created role one minute and abandoning it the next.

> *During a family therapy session Evan, aged 14, suddenly began to make dramatic swaying movements and strange howling sounds that were a parody of craziness. It was hard to judge Evan's relationship to his performance. Was he absorbed in his madness role in the way he might identify with one of his PlayStation avatars? Was he protesting? Performing a role does not entail a simple choice between pretence and sincerity.*

An Australian sorcerer who removes magical arrows from the bodies of people suffering from rheumatism knows that they are only pebbles taken from his mouth, according to the sociologist Michel Mauss, but his simulations are not simple matters of fraud: they are both voluntary and involuntary. 'The magician then becomes his own dupe, in the same way as an actor when he forgets that he is playing a role'.[17] This suggests a more plausible psychology of illness performance than a simplistic false-real dichotomy. If John sometimes believed his non-epileptic seizures were straightforward epilepsy, perhaps this was because he came to inhabit a role rather than merely playing it. If so, his behaviour probably did represent some reality, if not a cerebral discharge of the kind that causes epilepsy. Several people watched Sam pumping up his tyre and then slipping back into his wheelchair. We continued to believe that the appearance of disability was telling us something true about him. Little Rowena was undoubtedly communicating something through her limp. Her body was speaking.

Encountering the sick body-self

For the moment let us stay with the question of how the body speaks[18] rather than try to decipher what the body might be saying (which is what the next chapter will try to do). Imagine visiting a friend in hospital. She's listless, not her usual self, and her body speaks of illness. There is hospital paraphernalia all around the bed, and your usual way of being with her has been disturbed. A picture of illness, or rather of disease, holds you captive, making you wonder what to say, and you are unsure what messages are coming from her either in words or otherwise. In Gwyneth Lewis's *Hospital Odyssey* someone on the way towards an ill person sees 'fronded capillaries swamped by tumours, her arteries flowing with mud'.[19]

The situation would not be radically different if you were meeting a friend with a psychiatric diagnosis. It might then seem as though an almost visible essence called mental illness lay between you and the other person. A third scenario finds you even more unsure of yourself because your friend is looking unexpectedly happy when she is supposed to be critically ill.

> *As I remember her, 35-year-old Lori is sitting on a chair beside her hospital bed, cheerfully holding court with her parents and cousin. Her medical records describe a mysterious and painful illness, but whenever I meet her she seems well enough. Lori accepts medical help with a smile, only to reject it later.*

Lori's feelings are a mystery, which is disguised by a picture of disease. In such situations what we see easily gets translated into what we do not want to see, and then into something we refuse to see. I wonder if Lori does not really want to be helped but is responding to a duty that the sociologist Talcott Parsons recognises, to try to get well[20]. Any doubts her family have about Lori's illness are transformed into an eager interest in medical tests, as more and more normal results came in.

Much of the time a doctor views a body as an object and does not hear the body speaking. Doctors are protected from being challenged by another person's illness in several ways. Just as a military trainee knows that one of the expectations of a soldier is that he or she should be willing to shoot and to kill, so we as students already knew that the doctor must not be shocked by, or even humanly interested in bodies. We cultivated a psychic splitting that protected us from what would have either repelled or attracted us about a body in any other place. An enormous freezer-like chest in our dissecting room contained a grotesque tangle of formalin-soaked limbs, each with an identity tag attached to it. We studiously avoided any personal associations that these arms and legs might have, our required attitude being laconic detachment. I now see that this was an initiation into the objective posture we were supposed to adopt with living patients. My composure very occasionally faltered in the dissecting room, and it often did so later when a patient's illness impacted on me in spite of my professional self. In the intensive care unit, for example, there was always something eerie (for me) about the relentless sighing of a ventilator attached to a comatose patient. I had the same feeling when I met the sightless eyes of someone having an epileptic seizure. I remember being deeply disturbed when a woman's intracranial pressure rose dramatically just as I was questioning her about her neck and head pain. Her body became grotesquely contorted and her personality disappeared before my eyes.

Friends and family are more shockable than doctors, and less certain of how they should relate to an ill person. They do not usually look at a body with a diagnosing eye, although they sometimes do, and most of the time they are not concerned with assessing the 'realness' of illness, although they sometimes are. Often, they are hoping to connect with a person rather than a patient. From her own experience of cancer Deborah Orr advises us on how not to do this, giving us ten things not to say to someone who is ill.[21] One is 'You're looking well', which negates the person's performance of illness, as though to deny its reality. Another is 'You're looking terrible', which reinforces the identity of illness rather than offering an escape from it. I think a further problem with 'You're looking terrible' is that the body rather than the person is being seen. We need to find ways of using what we see as a means of understanding what the ill person sees.

An intuitive alternative to Deborah Orr's 'do nots' would be to suppress the speaker's feelings entirely, but in an encounter with someone else's ill-being it is impossible to efface one's self. When I am anywhere near the illness of someone I know, I feel myself getting dangerously close to things I normally need not face. The body itself is one of those familiar and yet unfamiliar things; death is another. Aspects of life that are usually hidden from view are all too visible in illness. I may see and smell more of a person's body than I want to. If this has become that individual's normality, I must enter it myself without flinching if I am to get close to his perspective. That does not mean I must deny my difficulties, because they may well mirror those of the other person. Glenda Fredman beautifully describes how talking about death with children and families can start from a position of admitting that I do not really know what to say.[22]

A dialogue is a meeting of bodies, and Rudebeck's recommendation of 'body-empathy' applies to doctors as it does to everyone.[23] Two brains are in the meeting, so that one body's behaviour is liable to trigger mirror neurons in the corresponding area of an observer's cerebral cortex.[24] You cannot be present to someone without being a physical presence. The doctor's or therapist's physical body sometimes stands for some figure from the past, for example a parent; and the patient's body can have similar significance for a clinician. These dynamics, called transference and countertransference in psychoanalysis, are unavoidable and need to be understood in any encounter with an ill person.

The bodily changes that diseases produce often obscure a person's individuality to the point where an entirely new individual seems to have been created. When someone with Parkinson's disease came into my clinic for the first time I often had the illusion that I knew that person. I am thinking of a man whose facial expression and posture and way of speaking forcibly reminded me of hundreds of other men I had met with the same diagnosis, so that I imagined I might understand his sense of humour before ever he spoke to me. Getting in touch with that person's individuality was hard work, especially because family members and professionals filled the room with their own more fluent personalities. In a personal encounter, as distinct from a clinical one, the focus is more on intentions than on biological facts. A crucial challenge is how to recognise someone's authentic personality.

A malingerer's efforts at self-expression are inauthentic, but those of a sincerely distressed person are truthful, whatever the underlying problem might be. The authenticity of symptoms hinges to a great degree on that of the person and authenticity is communicated as much through the body – through gestures and facial expressions and tone of voice – as through what is said. The critical importance of appearances generated a great deal of ambivalence for me in my role as a CFS/ME specialist, because my medical gaze was directed less towards objective facts than towards the person that I could see before me. Judging whether fatigue, for example, was out of the ordinary depended almost entirely on assessing what could be sensed or 'seen' of an individual's human qualities.[25] The hallmarks of malingering I identified earlier largely concern what the person says, which is how the credibility of a legal witness is supposed to be determined,[26] but police work presumably involves judging how genuine a suspect appears to be. The body speaks more eloquently than words in such situations.

Notes

1 Mechanic 1961
2 Goffman 1956/1990
3 Alonzo 1985
4 Griffith & Ryan 2015
5 Rumsey et al. 1982
6 Douglas 1966/1984
7 Clarke & James 2003
8 Dickson Wright 1955–56
9 Pearce 2004
10 Bass & Halligan 2014; Adetunji et al. 2006; Edens & Guy 2001
11 Asher 1951
12 See Lewis 1975; Mayou 2014
13 Miller 1978, p. 53
14 Broyard 1992, p. 45
15 For cross-cultural perspectives on malingering see Nijdam-Jones 2017; Bartholomew 1994; Trnka 2007
16 You will malinger better if you study research evidence e.g. Edens & Guy 2001; Nijdam-Jones 2017. See also How Psychologists Determine Whether Someone Is Faking Insanity. The Cut. 2017; Feb 1 www.thecut.com/2017/02/how-hard-is-it-to-fake-insanity.html
17 Mauss 1902/1972 p. 117–118
18 I owe this phrase to Griffith & Griffith 1994
19 Lewis 2010
20 Parsons 1964, Chapter 7
21 Guardian 18/4/2012 www.theguardian.com/lifeandstyle/2012/apr/18/10-things-not-say-when-ill
22 Fredman 1997
23 Rudebeck 2000
24 Whether to equate this directly with empathy is another question. See Lamma & Majdandžić 2015
25 See Ward 2015 b – 'The said and the unsaid: ambivalence in CFS/ME'. This was the kind of situation that the sociologist Robert Merton called sociological ambivalence ('incompatible normative expectations incorporated within a single role'), the expectations here being two kinds of practice, (a) as a science-based expert and (b) as a so-called 'healer' (Merton 1976 p. 6, see also Chapter 4, 'The Ambivalence of Physicians').
26 Janna, P. Determining the credibility of a witness (Excelerate v Cumberbatch). Lexisnexis blog, 28/1/2015 https://blogs.lexisnexis.co.uk/content/dispute-resolution/determining-the-credibility-of-a-witness-excelerate-v-cumberbatch

6

MEANINGS

'Every human cognitive reaction – perceiving, imagining, remembering, thinking and reasoning – [is] an effort after meaning', according to the experimental psychologist Frederick Bartlett.[1] Chapter 4 described how meanings are distilled from the firstness of ill-being. The following chapter was about the efforts a person must make to 'perform' symptoms in ways that are meaningful to others. This one explores meanings more directly.

From a disease perspective, biological signs have objective meanings that are entirely separate from the meanings that people attach to their experiences. It is true that my horse chestnut tree is diseased, whatever the tree may think. In illness, on the other hand, there is a two-way relationship between personal feelings and bodily processes. Illness is experienced through symptoms that can be physically explained, but interpreting the personal significance of illness goes beyond the body. Conversely, personal meanings have physical effects. These two aspects of illness are held together by beliefs. Viktor Frankl heard a man describe a dream predicting that he would be liberated on March 30 1945. When March 30 came without any sign of freedom the man became delirious, and died of typhus the following day.[2] The effects of stress on the immune system might perhaps explain the timing of this man's disease, which connects with physiological accounts of placebo effects, but the personal meanings of this episode also call for interpretation. Illness is an alloy of facts and values, making explanation and interpretation two sides of the same coin.

Beliefs

Later, I will be describing several people with multiple sclerosis (MS). Any sense of illness or wrongness they experience is a question of preference and belief – of values, or aesthetics – rather than of facts. Values collide with the biological facts in

MS, as they do in any medical situation. Conversely, feelings and meanings seem to influence the pathological process of MS.[3] Mental states certainly have effects on another neurological condition, dystonia, which causes unsightly and sometimes disabling spasms of muscles around the eyes or in the neck. The facts about dystonia are somewhat obscure, but it is often due to dysfunction of the brain's basal ganglia. When I was treating dystonic patients with botulinum toxin, I could see for myself how the needle occasionally stopped the symptoms instantaneously, long before the toxin's effects could have begun. On one occasion the patient improved to the same extent as with previous injections, which surprised and relieved me when I found later that the dose was far lower than it should have been. These were placebo effects. The anthropologist Daniel Moerman calls them meaning effects, because they are biological changes that are produced by the significance – the value – that a person attaches to a treatment ritual such as injection, or to the person who performs it. His review of the placebo literature leaves little doubt that placebos have physical effects outside the realm of imagination.[4]

In terms of Peirce's theory, any sign can be meaningful for someone, and personal beliefs are what often make the link. My patients would sometimes express strong beliefs about what had caused a fit, or a stroke, or a heart attack. They might be convinced that weakness of a limb was due to hard physical work, despite my clinical view of it as an attack of MS. Self-blame is often an emotive issue, usually on account of a habit of mind that is so deep-seated that it might be better thought of as a culturally-acquired habitus (particularly among mothers, in my experience) than an explicit belief. However, illness is a sign of divine action for many people across the world.

Daphne was a woman with MS who stuck to her opinion that her illness was a punishment from God, no matter what medical theories I suggested.

At one time I might have thought of non-medical ideas about causation as primitive and unhelpful but I have come to see them as natural efforts to reconcile bodily experiences with meanings. Strong opinions about biological explanations arise from an ill person's own beliefs about the action of the mind on the body and also from that person's assumptions about the beliefs of others. We know that symptoms are situated within our lives, and we are committed to taking responsibility for events wherever we can, but however much we theorise about bodies, souls, minds, life and death, none of us is sure how to describe our situation, or how it relates to illness. Philosophers' ideas about the way the body and the self are related rarely convince me, so it is not surprising that individuals who are living with the same dilemmas at close quarters hold beliefs that are inconsistent and self-contradictory. Uncertainties can become intense when we are overwhelmed by illness or when death is near.

Someone who attaches a particular meaning to symptoms or illness is not necessarily subscribing to a proposition in the way that a scientist works with an evidence-based hypothesis. The relationship between a person and a belief can be warmer than that. People hold to beliefs about illness - they may hold them dear – much as a person may live within a religious faith rather than theorizing about it.[5] Beliefs flow from the way different individuals have experienced the world. A person who holds to the view that her symptoms are caused by stress is very likely to reflect the common sense of individuals she has lived with and loved. For another person, the idea that the mind is connected in any way with bodily illness may fly in the face of a different common sense.

As a doctor I often thought it was my job to replace false accounts of illness with correct ones. I now see that I was resorting to a common sense that belonged to my own cultural and personal context, which led me to expect that contradictions and inconsistencies would eventually yield to the sword of truth. Had I come from a Chinese background my tolerance of contradiction might have been greater, making me more willing to allow different registers of meaning to co-exist.[6] No-one has a seamlessly consistent view of the world, which is why many people in western as well as eastern societies make use of western and traditional medicine simultaneously. People's ways of making sense of the world are not typically consistent from a logical point of view and nor are the beliefs that underpin them necessarily robust. There is a story about the physicist Nils Bohr having a horse-shoe nailed to a door. Asked if he really thought that it could bring him good luck he replied 'No, but I'm told that it's equally effective whether I believe in it or not'.

Explanation

A sick person's effort after meaning is a quest primarily for explanation, whether medical ('does this cough mean that I have cancer?'), psychological ('am I stressed?'), supernatural ('have I been cursed?') or philosophical ('why me?'). Even Job, when he questions God about his bodily affliction, is looking for an explanation.[7]

Signs and symbols

The rise of scientific medicine made illness something to be observed, classified and manipulated rather than understood in human terms. Victorian doctors searched the bodies of their patients for signs of disease, without much regard for feelings or thoughts. In their eyes, mental illness was as physical as any other kind, so that doctors looked for signs ('stigmata') of hysteria just as they looked for signs of typhoid. In semiotic terms they thought of a symptom as an *index*, which is a sign that indicates – points directly towards – what it represents.[8] A hysterical fit was an index of a brain state, just as a cough was an index of respiratory trouble. Today the physical aspect of psychological stress can be foregrounded in a similar way, so that a symptom such as nausea or palpitations is seen as an index of a physiological stress reaction. Wahid's paraplegia (p. 49) could be interpreted in psychological terms as a conversion disorder (p. 5), but MR studies show changes in conversion patients, making it possible to see their psychologically-based symptoms simply as an index of 'selective decreases in the activity of frontal and subcortical circuits'.[9]

Freud and his followers would often see a physical symptom as a symbol (rather than as an index). Wahid's paralysis below the waist could have symbolised sexual anxieties, and Elaine's blindness (p. 48) might have symbolised an inner darkness of some kind. Freudian theory says that a physical symptom can replace feelings that would otherwise be intolerable. This would be a way of explaining why Lori (p. 53) seemed so unconcerned about her mysterious illness.

Freud has been regarded as a mechanist at heart, a 'biologist of the mind'[10], but he never gave a mechanistic account of how a symbolic process could produce physical symptoms. Ferenczi, one of the early psychoanalysts, almost did so. He suggested that when words are lacking, for example in the midst of a traumatic experience, unspeakable feelings might 'materialise' as a sort of bodily precipitate.[11] More recently, a phenomenon called body memory has been postulated as a consequence of psychological trauma.[12] A patient of mine had a sensation in the elbow that was, to him, a symptom of a physical illness. He casually mentioned to me that the feeling reminded him of 'when our child died in my arms'.

Medical objectivism

Foster Kennedy, a neurologist the 1920s, wrote that 'psychological interpretations are just figure-skating on the surface of the problem; the aim should always be the examination of defects of structure'.[13] At that time Freudian concepts were in the ascendancy, but in today's neurology Kennedy's attitude prevails: the pendulum has swung back from psychological to biological modes of explanation.[14] Contemporary medicine has been producing an ever-widening repertoire of medical tests that seem to reduce the need to ask patients questions even about their bodies, let alone their feelings.

The ill person is being silenced, once again, by technology, but when biomedicine disregards the psychological context it often has to make do with very skimpy explanations for symptoms. The label 'CFS/ME' describes a diagnostic pattern, and it is no more an explanation for the physical symptoms than migraine is for headache, or schizophrenia for hallucinations. 'Ah yes' says Richard Asher's imaginary doctor to a patient with an inflamed tongue. 'You have glossitis'. 'Thank you doctor' says the patient. 'It's all right now I know what it is'.[15]

> Gwen complains of overwhelming fatigue, and constantly suffers from what she calls 'brain fog', along with disturbed sleep and pains in her joints, muscles, spine and head. She wonders if her illness is a reaction to the years in which she has been super-healthy, super-competent, and super-busy, simultaneously organising a dry-cleaning business, a family and a divorce.

Gwen crashed down from the heights of success and became physically ill. Her story is a familiar one in the world of CFS/ME. It is reminiscent of the character-type Freud named 'wrecked by success',[16] but Gwen would have been angry if I had offered this or any other purely psychological narrative as an explanation for her symptoms. She would have been right to be annoyed, because even if the Freudian story contained a grain of truth it would not make her physical sufferings and disability sufficiently intelligible to her. The fatigue of CFS/ME is publicly described as 'debilitating',[17] but Gwen would find it difficult to accept that she was being physically debilitated by anything connected with personal meanings.

Suppose Gwen had come across the following recent headline: 'CFS is no longer a mystery – it is caused by biofilm bacteria'. She would probably have taken this idea more seriously than Freud's, but even if biofilm bacteria provided a viable biological explanation, which I doubt, it would not have made her symptoms any easier to understand. At a bodily level Gwen's brain fog and fatigue and diffuse pain would not have been cured by antiseptic spray, and nor would bacteriology help her see connections between physical symptoms and personal life.

Offering biofilm bacteria as a totalising explanation is an example of medical objectivism, or medical materialism as William James called it. He mocked the assumption that Saint Paul's activities could be 'explained away' as a discharging lesion of the occipital cortex or George Fox's spiritual quest as a disordered colon.[18] Medical objectivism looks for clinical diagnoses that explain creativity (Samuel Johnson, Emily Dickinson) tyranny (Hitler) and philosophical brilliance (Marcus Aurelius).[19] The use of neuroimaging to explain human experience is a form of medical objectivism.

Medical objectivism is an ideology that doctors and patients often share. It explains the contemporary pressure to diagnose. Siri Hustvedt, by no means an arch-objectivist, describes her efforts to explain some abnormal feelings she has had in her limbs for years. First, she ignores them, then wonders about MS and consults a doctor, who reassures her. The doctor diagnoses peripheral neuropathy, which is an often-benign condition that is difficult to prove or disprove. Hustvedt wonders if her presumptive neuropathy has been caused by a drug she is taking. Her doctor is doubtful, but discovers that it is a possible side-effect (many drugs occasionally cause neuropathy). She then suggests an entirely different explanation for her symptoms: migraine. Her doctor does not believe migraine causes this kind of thing but, says Hustvedt, 'later, I discovered he was wrong'.[20] Despite her confidence, there are no definite criteria in this story for what is 'wrong' or 'right'. The symptoms come to roost, finally, on a very questionable medical diagnosis. Medical explanation seems to be a necessary terminus, and yet all it achieves is to substitute one form of uncertainty – 'I'm not sure what these symptoms mean' – for another: 'This might or might not be migraine'.

Medical objectivism gives 'how' precedence over 'why', by implying that the meaning of illness is entirely contained in its physical mechanisms. Precisely why symptoms like Gwen's come about is ignored. On the other hand, when 'why' takes precedence over 'how' we have thin explanations of the 'wrecked by success' variety. Physical explanation has then been abandoned as though a psychological account were sufficient. Stories like that of Lisa Steen, a young GP, published after her death, fuel the desire for medical explanations of symptoms. After a combination of unusual symptoms and negative tests a psychological explanation was assumed. Her identity as someone with 'health anxiety' made it less and less possible for her to be heard, physically examined, and investigated until cancer of the kidney was finally discovered.[21]

When I remove my sock I am hoping that the doctor will inspect my foot, not my soul, so it is as well for doctors not to be distracted from their primary task of diagnosing disease. Wittgenstein was wary of the Freudian mode of explanation because symbols, analogies and metaphors have a beguiling power that outstrips their ability to explain what people are saying or doing in the real world.[22] A similar position inspired Susan Sontag's attack on the notion that nineteenth century 'consumption' (which generally meant pulmonary tuberculosis) was metaphorically expressive of romantic decadence, or that HIV/AIDS somehow represented moral decay in the late 20th century. On similar grounds Barbara Ehrenreich rejects the idea that cancer in any sense embodies the sufferer's personal failures.[23]

Just as doctors can be held captive by psychology, so psychologists can be seduced by neuroscience, rather than attending to the non-physical sources of illness. Problems arise when the quest for either a physical or psychological diagnosis is a distraction from what is most relevant and most meaningful to the sick person. To say, as medical objectivists do, that every variety of illness, from cancer to CFS/ME, has a biological mechanism is a truism. It contributes little to the understanding of illness, and nor does the equally vacuous proposition that psychological factors are always relevant. When doctors, sometimes along with their patients, become preoccupied with distinguishing physical from psychological explanations they are often missing the point. Perhaps George Fox's colon did influence his spiritual life but the mind – or, if you like, the spirit – also influences the guts. Illness has multiple, complex origins that naïve medical objectivism cannot take into account.

Medical explanation reaches its endpoint when a doctor declines to diagnose someone's ache, or dizziness, or fatigue as an illness, saying that these are 'normal' experiences. Normality has no explanation, no cause. If the patient feels ill he will be disappointed. A psychological formulation such as 'health anxiety' could offer a crumb of comfort. 'Hypochondriasis' might be a preferable label because it would be a medical diagnosis and hence provide a meaningful identity, however shabby this may seem in the eyes of others.[24] When medical explanation defines the boundary of illness, it leaves many people with nowhere to go when they are troubled.

Psychological explanation

Lucy Johnstone, a clinical psychologist, identifies a sharp dichotomy. Either 'you have a medical disease with primarily biological causes', she says, or else 'your problems are an understandable emotional response to your life circumstances'.[25] Many people, including doctors and psychologists, see psychological explanations in this way, as logically incompatible with a 'medical' (i.e. biological) account. A headline about unexplained chronic pain triumphantly pronounced that 'Neurophysiology explains the unexplained',[26] as though some biological finding could strike a decisive blow in a zero–sum contest between physical and psychological explanations.

The 'widely divergent and hotly contested beliefs' associated with CFS/ME, as with other contested diagnoses, create a political battleground in which a strictly biological narrative is promoted forcefully, and sometimes even violently. People with contested diagnoses often see psychological explanation as a threat. The danger is real. Many of our patients and research participants had encountered a GP who 'didn't believe in it'. Some doctors would agree with a journalist who inferred from the results of a trial on CFS/ME that the best treatment was to 'get out for a nice walk once in a while and maybe see a shrink'.[27]

> *Henry was a man in search of a physical explanation for his neurological symptoms. He was angered by my enquiries about the psychological context and as he was leaving the room turned to me and loudly said that his problems had 'nothing to do with the time when I was trapped in the burning building'.*

Given Henry's non-specific symptoms I found it hard to believe that they were not connected with this traumatic experience. I think he worried that if I accepted such an explanation, I would not be believing that he was ill.

In both medicine and psychiatry there is continuing tension between a disease-oriented view and a psychologically-based approach. Ancient Hippocratic medicine's emphasis on bodily balance was a reaction against the idea that a symptom was a sign from the gods. Technological medicine in the nineteenth century arose in a similar spirit. Its body-centred objectivism led to what the sociologist Nicholas Jewson described as the 'disappearance of the sick-man'.[28] One of Freud's great contributions was to show that certain symptoms can only be understood by listening carefully to what the sufferer has to say about them. He turned the focus back towards a person's feelings and thoughts, so that the sick man (and woman) got a speaking part in the drama of medicine. In the 1950s, the development of antipsychotic drugs and other powerful medical approaches to mental stress seemed to make the patient's voice once again marginal if not irrelevant, which provoked anti-psychiatrists such as RD Laing into producing family-based accounts of mental disorders.[29] Psychiatry today is heavily influenced by recent advances in neuroscience, triggering a new wave of critical psychologists and anti-psychiatrists.[30]

The same tensions are mirrored outside the orthodox professional world. On the one hand there is plenty of breezy psychologising that sees meaning everywhere, as in this account of rheumatoid arthritis from the internet: 'The degree of seriousness [of the arthritis] is relative to the degree of emotional, mental, and spiritual blockage. Generally, if you suffer from rheumatoid arthritis, you are very self-critical . . .'.[31] On the other hand, there is a plethora of unorthodox medical explanations and remedies to be explored, for example, in the magazine 'What Doctors Don't Tell You'.[32]

Sociological explanation

Illness and diagnosis are spoken of as 'things' that 'belong' to one individual, but if several people in a community have similar symptoms, we should surely look for explanations within the group. We need sociological imagination, as the American sociologist C Wright Mills called it,[33] to lift ourselves up to an altitude where we see groups rather than individuals and 'public issues' (in Mills' words) rather than 'personal troubles'. A health problem that looks unique to an individual can be viewed as a social symptom. When I was a trainee doctor my boss advised me to give people simple explanations ('It's the brain' or 'it's the heart') rather mini-lectures. If I had said 'it's society' (or in a political vein, 'I blame the government'), I would sometimes have been correct.

> *15-year-old Jordan is anxious and erratic.*[34] *From age 10 to 13 she witnessed violent conflicts between her parents Shelley and George, who separated two years ago. Shelley, who now looks after Jordan along with her two other children, is heavily in debt and receiving long-term antidepressant drugs through her GP. Alcohol triggered the violence that ended Shelly and George's marriage. George is attending a liver clinic at the local hospital.*

Medical diagnoses abound in Jordan's family: autism spectrum disorder (ASD) and also obsession compulsion disorder (OCD) for Jordan herself; depression for Shelley; and alcoholic liver disease for George. New meanings – new explanations – open up, however, when the family is seen in its societal context. These are not just personal troubles, but also public issues. Many families in the city where Jordan lives have had similar experiences of abuse and poverty, and a disproportionate number receive multiple psychiatric diagnoses. Gender is another public issue for Jordan and Shelley: women are almost twice as likely as men to report severe symptoms of common mental disorders in the UK. [35] George's alcohol is also a public issue. The psychiatric labels used in Jordan's family are helpful in some circumstances, just as the label 'cirrhosis of the liver' is a necessary way of describing George, but these diagnoses are not sufficient explanations of the troubles they purport to explain. They are terrible simplifications (see p. 20), because they make it possible to deny or at least to minimise the complexities that sociological imagination reveals.

Families live between the poles of personal troubles and public issues. Besides genes, families share belief systems and contexts and ways of being that influence the strategies that different individuals adopt at times of crisis. In a family as in any social context the word 'explanation' only becomes fully credible when it includes everything that influences symptoms. An explanation should not bind an individual into a chain of causes and effects because most elements in a system are linked to one another in more complex ways, with causes and effects often influencing one another. A systemic description often decentres the person whom medicine identifies as the bearer of a diagnosis, so that the problem's roots in immediate relationships and in wider social processes become clearer. A sociological explanation has some of the shortcomings of medical explanation, however, since no mechanistic account encompasses all the personal meanings that illness can have.

Explanation and professional power

Modes of explanation are a political issue within the professional world because they define the spheres of influence that sociologists call 'jurisdictions'.[36] Health professionals have an investment in looking for pathology in individuals like Jordan and her two parents, just as corporations that supply health products and services have financial investments in illness. Non-biological explanations of illness challenge biomedicine's right to interpret distress. The criticism of doctors by psychologists and vice versa reflects competitive tensions between professional jurisdictions.

Medical specialists are strong defenders of their jurisdiction. In the last hundred years the number of specialists and specialisms has steadily increased in the US, Britain and across the world. Specialists owe much of their status, power and income to their ability to produce medical explanations for symptoms. A specialist who judged that most patients did not need a medical diagnosis would soon lose credibility. When someone referred a patient to me as a Parkinson's disease specialist, I would not have been human if I didn't get satisfaction at times from coming up with some arcane alternative to the diagnosis of plain Parkinson's. Investigations add to the medicalising effects of specialist diagnosis. They make doctors feel under a legal as well as a moral obligation 'to leave no stone unturned'. The medical plough could grind on almost forever if no stone was to be left unturned.

One way of extending medical jurisdiction across a person's life is to apply additional diagnostic labels, known in medical jargon as co-morbidities. Jordan currently has two diagnoses, ASD and OCD, but she has also been assessed for attention deficit hyperactivity disorder (ADHD) because of her restlessness, and other suggested labels have included 'pathological demand avoidance', and 'emerging borderline personality disorder'. Many adolescents and adults carry two or more concurrent psychiatric labels. It would be fanciful to imagine that Jordan has succumbed, coincidentally, to several distinct medical diseases. Jordan's multiplicity of labels demonstrates the difficulty in stretching diagnostic categories across the complexities of her life.

Medical jurisdiction can also be extended by pathologising a person's supposed normality. A healthy-feeling person can be diagnosed with a 'latent' disease such as pre-diabetes. Symptoms, and some defects of the body's structure or function, can appear to be unfinished versions or 'formes frustes' of medical conditions, as if a disease is about to release its frustration by bursting out from beneath the skin. Normalities are also medicalized through genetics. Genes can be invoked as explanations for human situations as diverse as obesity, alcoholism, risk-taking behaviour and back pain.[37] Yet another way of widening the reach of medical explanation is to relax the boundaries of a diagnosis so that more people are eligible for it.

If all else fails in the effort to describe things in medical terms, a problem can always be labelled as 'medically unexplained'. This gives medicine limitless explanatory power, since everything in the universe either is or is not 'medically explained', just as everything is either astrologically explained or astrologically unexplained. As I said in Chapter 3 (p. 24–25), ways of knowing illness are allied to ways of not-knowing. On the internet CFS/ME is often described as mysterious, but this might be simply because it cannot be neatly described in medical terms.[38]

Not many ill people are conscious of being tossed around in a political pinball machine. Patients and their doctors are usually unaware of why they are the winners or losers in struggles for power. Doctors would be more useful to their patients if they could appreciate the social dimensions of meaning, just as many ill people would get better more quickly if they were gifted with sociological imagination.

Interpretation

The main goals of biological and of psychological explanation are therapeutic. Even a sociological explanation is often intended, ultimately, to emancipate people: I would like Jordan and her family to somehow gain more power over their situation than is possible within a medical framework. Not all kinds of understanding seek to change a situation, however. I often observed how a convulsion or an attack of dizziness could shake someone existentially as well as physically. Such feelings needed to be interpreted within the person's life world. The task of interpretation includes but goes far beyond the realm of explanation.

Clive, a man whose legs were paralysed by MS, told me that one of the worst things about his disability was that when he was out in his wheelchair with his wife he couldn't 'stand up for her'.

Clive had lost the ability to physically stand, but I thought he was also mourning the loss of what he saw as a man's protective power.[39] Paraplegia was a meaningful symbol, without being an explanation for anything other than the way he saw the world. Clive's ability to interpret his own experience was probably useful to him in his effort to make sense of his feelings. It gave me a better chance of empathising with him, and also of identifying what he felt himself to need.

The distinction between explanation and interpretation is real and necessary, but not clear-cut. The two terms are often used interchangeably in medicine, as when a pathologist interprets a specimen, or a doctor interprets a clinical picture. All causal explanations are interpretations, I admit, but the reverse is not true. Understanding a situation is worthwhile even when there is no agenda to explain or change it. Interpretation touches on personal knowledge that is meaningless from an explanatory point of view, and discloses the shadows of what may only be knowable symbolically.

Explanations are always in some sense normative. Gwen's fatigue, pain, and sleeplessness might be considered by her doctor to be 'only normal'. If symptoms are normal in this sense there is nothing to explain, which is to say that Gwen is not 'really' ill. This leaves her with a sense of ill-being that appears to be meaningless. It would be tempting to say that Jordan's behavior is a normal reaction to social stresses. Saying this would not relieve Jordan of her feelings. The kind of interpretation I am recommending will not deny the reality of a person's experience and will seek to tease out layers of meaning that are beyond the scope of mechanistic explanation. Interpretation is achieved through open dialogue and resembles the processes that are known academically as ethnography, or phenomenology, or hermeneutics.[40]

The level of meaning I am working towards here is very personal, and a clinician can only dimly perceive it from the outside. Let me be the unreliable witness to some experiences of my own. When I was a teenager, I had a short episode of suddenly being unable to march. I was part of a military display in which the whole school was watching our squad compete in the annual drill competition. When the drums rolled and the order came – 'Quiiiiick march!' –, my right leg came out along with my right arm, instead of alternating smoothly. The result was a highly unmilitary waddle and our chances of winning were ruined. Years later, as a neurologist, I would have diagnosed this as a kind of 'hysterical' conversion similar to Wahid's.

In these situations it is the body that speaks. At the time it was not clear to me what my body was saying, just as Wahid was mystified by his paraplegia. I now think that I was feeling ambivalent, torn between the contradictory goals of escaping from something I detested and demonstrating prowess within it. This was an 'unspeakable dilemma'.[41] One would not need to be a Freud to think that Henry's nonchalant remark about his house fire was evidence of a connection between his symptoms and something almost unspeakable.

Functional symptoms attract interpretations, but attaching similar meanings to diagnoses such as cancer and HIV/AIDS seems highly questionable. Is this because there are some conditions that can be interpreted meaningfully and others that cannot? If so, which are the sorts of illnesses that we must not interpret? How would we know when to stop suggesting that symptoms have meanings? Whilst making my first application for a university chair I had an experience that shook my confidence in distinguishing 'organic' from 'functional' illness. I had feelings of dread (how must I act to be credible?); excitement (would this place be my future?); and guilt (how could I expect my family to move from the home they loved?). My body spoke: the left foot became inflamed and swollen with cellulitis. The air of confidence and competence I needed was blown away by my amateurish crutch-walking. (Needless to say, I didn't get the job). Cellulitis was probably an index of physiological stress, which can radically affect the body's immune reactivity, but my puffy, painful foot was also saying something else. It made me lame in the eyes of the world but at the same time somehow embodied an inner lameness.

Cause or effect? When the body speaks this is not the right question. In ill-ness the body speaks to me, and also through me. The world often wrongly imagines that a person with the tremor of Parkinson's disease is anxious. However, I sometimes wonder if an individual with parkinsonian tremor might come to see herself as others see her, and hence risk of becoming the fumbling, anxious person that other people think they see. Physical symptoms do some-times insinuate themselves into the personality to the point where boundaries between normal and pathological, between voluntary and involuntary (or between symbol and index) become blurred. A cancer affecting the face or voice, or a dental abscess, or even a trivial problem such as blocked sinuses almost inevitably becomes part of the way one experiences oneself at the same time as affecting how one is experienced by others. The involuntary move-ments of Huntington's disease and cerebral palsy sometimes seem to have been willed, so that it would be rash to dismiss them as meaningless. I have often watched a spiralling movement of the arm begin as though controlled by a random neurological mechanism and then evolve into a gesture that means something in its conversational context. One young man's side-to-side head movements had a neurological description (dystonia), but I also thought of them as conveying a message that I read as refusal or denial of something he had told me about her past: 'No, no'.

The American psychoanalyst and neurologist Smith Ely Jelliffe[42] described a young man with spasms of respiratory muscles due to encephalitis lethargica (EL), a brain infection that occurred in epidemics from 1917 to 1940. Jelliffe's patient dreamt that he entered a brothel in which he watched as his friend 'puffed and grunted . . . (just like I do)'. According to Jelliffe the man's involuntary eye movements were 'sufficient to inform the ego of its release from danger' and 'the puffing was therefore held to be a coitus equivalent, which releases the It impulse and . . . saves the patient from anxiety sufficiently intense to drive him to the feared thing, total castration, i.e. the death wish – suicide'. This sort of account, based on Freudian theory, is easy to mock but not, I think, because its attitude to interpretation is intrinsically wrong. The fusion of meanings with bodies reaches its apotheosis in the process psychoanalysts call projection. A person's body has the ability to evoke emotions, and hence to communicate with another person – another body. An abnormal body may be feared, which is part of the way stigma operates. A body may also represent something or someone to another individual, as in transference.

The merits and the menace of meaning

What good is done by interpreting symptoms as meaningful? And when is it useful to think of symptoms as meaningless? I have already touched on the negative moral overtones that can attach to cancer and TB. Self-blame was very often in the background when patients insisted, as they often did, that it was no accident that they had contracted MS, or Parkinson's disease.

Moira, the mother of a young woman with Huntington's disease knew logically that genetic mutations are nobody's fault and that it was her husband who had unwittingly brought Huntington's into the family, but she still constantly said 'I blame myself'.

Interpreting someone's behaviour as the meaningless effect of illness is helpful if, for example, it saves a child with ADHD from being blamed for being merely naughty. Such conditions are meaningless acts of fate, not metaphors or symbols of anything. No-one is to blame. Rain falls on the just and the unjust.

A diagnosis has the helpful effect of reducing both blame and its close relative shame. I have often encouraged family members in their wish to think that 'It's not him, it's his Huntington's...'; 'it's his Alzheimer's that makes him like that'. We would always insist that there is nothing shameful about epilepsy, or involuntary movements, or mobility problems. If psychological derangement seems shameful a medical diagnosis will be preferred. Without a medical diagnosis, fatigue will look like weakness of the will and depression will be seen as self-pity, because of the negative connotations of psychological explanation.

Diagnosis externalises the problem. It is often valuable from a therapeutic point of view to get away from the idea that your symptoms are integral to you, as though their badness was your badness. Imagining cancer as something pervasive, infiltrating one's bloodstream and organs, easily leads to a sense of powerlessness, as though the whole person, rather than just one part of the body, has become malignant. People are often encouraged by seeing a disease as something external. A split between one's self and one's disease turns illness into an object that can be fought against and conquered. Patients often talked about 'my Parkinson's disease' or 'this wretched multiple sclerosis' as hostile presences in their lives, and many books have been written about overcoming ME, fibromyalgia, depression and many other illnesses.[43] Families are able to deal with someone's dangerous compulsion not to eat more easily when it is externalised as 'Ali's anorexia'.

Ali was a teenager diagnosed with an anorexia. She resisted efforts to externalise her situation in this way. She said she pictured her problem as a virus that had become an inseparable part of herself. This gave Ali the feeling that she had no alternative but to restrict her eating so as to achieve the body shape she desired.

Ali might have been spared much suffering if she had viewed her anorexia as a disease-like entity that was alien to her.

A final and very menacing aspect of meaning is that it unsettles relationships. Disease is firm ground for patients, doctors and everyone. We know how to respond, or we think we do, when someone has cancer. Illness without obvious disease is more of a challenge. If physical symptoms 'do not add up' it may seem as if something is being left unsaid, which causes anxiety. The stigma that some people experience in relation to psychological distress is one reason for this, and doubt about whether an illness is 'real' illness makes it more difficult to relate to a person warmly. In meetings with patients like Lori, I needed to be able to think of them as in some sense ill, however incongruous their stories might be. I am describing a dynamic that goes in both directions because people with ambiguous illness stories are understandably wary of how they will be received once a psychological cause has been touted.

Despite the risks, meanings need not be a threat and are never an irrelevance. The positive value of interpretation is very apparent in systemic narrative therapy. Individuals and families often experience relief when, for example, the medical problem is no longer the default focus of a conversation. They are sometimes shocked but also relieved when 'the problem' is seen as something different from 'the patient'.[44] The doctor and the family can see illness as meaningful without having to share the same theories about the mind and the brain, or the same beliefs.

Notes

1 Bartlett 1932
2 Frankl 1964, p. 74–5
3 Mohr et al. 2004
4 Moerman 2002
5 Good 2007; the idea of preference is retained in the German word 'belieben' but has almost gone from 'belief' (see Smith 1998, Chapter 2), although we do have 'cherished beliefs'
6 In comparative studies of people with Chinese and with American cultural backgrounds, Chinese people were more likely than Americans to use a dialectical rather than an either/or strategy to resolve conflicts and to conduct arguments and appeared less wedded to the principle of non-contradiction (Peng & Nisbett 1999)
7 The Bible, Book of Job
8 Merrell 2001; Peirce 1931–1966 Vol 2 para 228
9 See Vuilleumier 2005
10 Sulloway 1979
11 Ferenczi 1926
12 Van der Kolk 2014
13 Kennedy 1926
14 Today's *Journal of Neurology, Neurosurgery and Psychiatry* contains little psychiatry and almost no references to psychodynamic theories. In the 1920s, as the *Journal of Neurology and Psychopathology*, it often included work based around psychoanalytic ideas
15 Asher 1972 p. 55
16 Freud 1914–1916
17 See for example Dinos et al. 2009; Fukuda et al. 1994; Times Online January 25 2010 www.thetimes.co.uk/article/me-a-debilitating-illness-with-no-known-cure-zpkv6t62cw2
18 James 1905 p. 13
19 Johnson: Sacks 1992; Dickinson: William Nicholson. Guardian 1/4/17 A Quiet Passion won't solve the mystery of Emily Dickinson – but does the truth matter?; Hitler: Coolidge et al. 2007; Marcus Aurelius: Duggan & Duggan 2006, Chapter 5a p. 33
20 Hustvedt (2011, p. 152) does simultaneously consider other, non-physical explanations for her symptoms. Porochista Khakpour's illness narrative is a similar but more complex odyssey that takes her from doctor to doctor in search of explanations for symptoms that include, but are perhaps not confined to, those of Lyme disease. Medical explanation always seems to be just round the corner, and often appears as the arbiter of realness (Khakpour 2018)
21 Steen, L. The wilderness of the medically unexplained BMJ Opinion 25/8/2016 https://blogs.bmj.com/bmj/2016/08/25/lisa-steen-the-wilderness-of-the-medically-unexplained/

22 Bouveresse 1995
23 Sontag 1978; Ehrenreich 2009
24 Cantor & Fallon 1996
25 Johnstone 2006 [In the quote I have substituted 'medical' for 'psychiatric']
26 Williams and Johnson 2011
27 Hotly contested', a quote from NICE 2007; violence: see Hawkes 2011; GPs: Saunders 2015; 'nice walk . . . ': Liddle, R. (The Spectator), November 2 2015. Let's just admit that chronic fatigue syndrome is not actually a chronic illness. https://blogs.spectator.co.uk/2015/11/lets-just-admit-that-chronic-fatigue-syndrome-is-not-actually-a-chronic-illness/
28 See Jewson 1976 for a historical account of how technological medicine silences the person
29 Laing 1960; Laing & Esterston 1964/1970; Sedgwick 1982
30 Fox et al. 2009; Nightingale & Cromby 2001
31 Bourbeau, L (undated). Metaphysical Definitions of 20 Illnesses/Diseases/Disorders.www.ecoutetoncorps.com/en/resources/metaphysical-definitions-20-illnessesdiseasesdisorders/
32 What Doctors Don't Tell You https://www.wddty.com/
33 Mills 1959
34 This story combines three different situations from my clinical work, with details altered to ensure anonymity
35 NHS Digital, 2016
36 Abbott 1988
37 Obesity: Choquet & Meyre 2011; alcoholism: National Institute on Alcohol Abuse and Alcoholism Genetics of alcohol use disorder https://www.niaaa.nih.gov/alcohol-health/; risk-taking behavior: Bell 2009; back pain: Williams AT et al. 2013
38 Rantzen, E. 2000
39 Arthur Kleinman (1988, p.41) describes a man with non-organic leg paralysis saying 'I never have been able to stan, stan, stand up on my own two feet before my, my, my father.'
40 The signs that explanations seek can often be quantified, as when rapid loss of weight is more predictive of cancer than the gradual loss of a couple of pounds. Whenever meanings within the field of interpretation seem to be measurable they pass into the domain of explanation, e.g. when someone discloses a belief that is strong enough to cause a low mood
41 See Griffith & Griffith 1994; Griffith & Ryan 2015; Showalter 1997; Hinton & Lewis-Fernández 2010; Furst 2002
42 Jelliffe 1925
43 E.g. Natelson 2008
44 See Ward et al. 2011 on medical applications of systemic therapy

PART II

Recovery

7

POSSIBILITIES

This chapter is about ways of being not ill, or of being less ill. What is it that people turn towards, or hope for, in times of illness? What are the possibilities? Health is a misleading concept, because it tends to suggest a standard image of wellness. There is no single way of getting better. Ill-being generates different needs in different individuals. In an exploration of possibilities, the notion of health is not necessarily helpful because it is a state that can only be achieved under specific, objective conditions and that for at least some of us is an impossible ideal. Less disease-bound words such as wellness, well-being and flourishing are useful. They mirror the character of ill-being, which does have a medical form but which merges almost imperceptibly with other versions of distress. However, all words for wellness have disadvantages. They often sound unduly static, rather like the traditional Christian image of heaven where everyone is resting beside the glassy sea. The difference between a static and a dynamic view of wellness is captured, or rather entangled, in the word 'better'. When I reassured a patient that he was better, meaning that he had improved, his wife was very indignant because she knew that he still had problems. 'Better' in her sense was the end of the illness story; 'better' to me was a moment in a process, or a milestone on a journey, or an orientation towards positive possibilities.

The idea of recovery generates similar misunderstandings. Recovery is sometimes a synonym for health, so that 'fully recovered' can mean 'completely healthy', but here I shall be depicting recovery as a process rather than an endpoint. Chronic physical illnesses call for a recovery process whereby well-being is sustained ('recovered') even though injuries persist or worsen. There is a form of recovery that is available even when one is dying. DW Winnicott's prayer is: 'Oh God! May I be alive when I die!'.[1]

The concept of recovery has roots in the experiences of alcoholics (in Alcoholics Anonymous), drug abusers, and 'survivors' of mental health services, all of whom want above all to recover the right and the ability to live as autonomous human beings. Patricia Deegan, a woman diagnosed with schizophrenia in her teens, says: 'Those of us who have been diagnosed are not objects to be acted upon. We are fully human subjects who can act and in acting, change our situation. We are human beings and we can speak for ourselves'.[2] People with physical disabilities make identical claims and anyone who retrieves a right or regains autonomy is recovering something – is a recovering person - just as anyone who has been held back either by impairments, by services or by the environment is in a real sense disabled.

The movement from illness towards something better has the form of a narrative.[3] A narrative perspective gives structure and meaning to illness, but it has limitations. An illness narrative turns a patient into an actor, making some experiences appear more controllable than they are. The narrative perspective also risks paradoxically diminishing the status of personal meanings while appearing to extol them, which happens when someone's story is regarded as a harmless but irrelevant nostrum ('if it works for you, that's fine'). Meanings cannot be marginalized in this way. Another problem is that stories always privilege what the narrator is willing and able to say. Most of the illness narratives I have come across are short on gory details. Who wants to hear about a runny nose, let alone a cancerous prostate? Writers often also seem to be reticent about, or oblivious to, their pre-illness stories, with all their potential traumas and ambiguities.

An illness narrative is often presented as a journey, a well-worn metaphor that can be carried too far. The journey image suggests that the traveller can decide where to go, which is hardly true if you are having a bout of gastroenteritis. A modern hospital resembles an airport, but you do not 'take' your journey through its endless queues, security checks, cancellations and revolving doors - it takes you. Gwyneth Lewis describes this beautifully from the point of view of a sufferer's wife, in *Hospital Odyssey* (which is more Dante than Homer)[4]. Another problem is that the idea of a journey invests too much in an imagined future. If motor neuron disease is slowly paralysing you, the journey's destination is death, so that you need a different image for the positive movements that can take place even in terminal situations. The journey of illness passes through a constantly changing landscape. An ill person is a nomad, always looking for better pastures but obliged somehow to make some sort of life along the way.

The journey's character depends on three interdependent factors. First there are images of health – standard, objective descriptions of what might count as well-being. The corollary of any such picture is a list of observable needs. Secondly there are personal needs, or desires, that cannot be so easily described because they arise from the subjectivity of ill-being. Standard definitions hardly seem to apply to incurable illness, and still less to an impending death, and yet in these situations there are needs, and there are positive possibilities of a sort. There are good deaths, and bad ones.[5] Thirdly, pictures of well-being and of personal needs create the directions in which an ill person will move. Some aim straight for a chosen goal, some meander towards unknown territory, and others circle endlessly around a single position.

Pictures of health

It is hard to have a picture of wellness when you are ill. Illness feels like the col-lapse of normality, but what is normal? Can it be defined in some standard way? The WHO's 1948 constitution defined health as 'a state of complete physical, mental and social well-being'.[6] This definition has the virtue of insisting that health combines three dimensions of human life rather than settling on a single one, as medicine often does. Viewing health as a physical state, a 'silence of the organs',[7] is a disease-centred concept that can make little sense of ill-being as a human experience. A solely psychological or spiritual concept of wellness has some appeal, on the other hand, given that many people seem able to live well despite extra-ordinary physical impairments. But if you could will yourself to be well, illness would be a symptom of character weakness. 'I don't do illness', one woman assured me. She had an air of brisk healthiness, in sharp contrast to the sickly-looking teen-age daughter she had brought to see me. The point seemed to be that her daughter's illness was a personal defect. A purely social image of health is also plausible, as seen among the well-nourished, well-clad farm children of Soviet propaganda, but such a picture leaves out the self-oriented aspect of illness and wellness. The WHO's three-dimensional definition is implausible given that no-one, surely, has ever been in a state of 'complete physical, mental and social well-being'.[8]

A more practical approach than the WHO's ambitious definition might be to define the needs that people experience in illness. Fatigue, nausea, anxiety and depression are things we want to be rid of and that we struggle against. Somewhere in us is the need to hold on to life, which is why obituaries so often describe someone's 'long battle with illness'. These basic needs easily translate into a quest for remedies, and in acute illness they form a clear hierarchy. Actions must be taken first to avoid death (resuscitation) and then to maintain life (fluids, nutrition, preventive nursing etc). A third priority, after those immediate needs have been attended to, is to attack the cause of illness, for example by treating infection with antibiotics or by clipping an artery that is bleeding into the brain. These correspond to the bottom layers in a hierarchy of needs devised by the American psychologist Abraham Maslow.[9] They apply as well to geese and ants as to people, but human well-being must also satisfy more personal needs.

One problem with Maslow's hierarchy is its rigidity, which breaks down in practice. The top level, self-actualisation, is both the effect and the cause of the level below it, which is self-esteem, just as the two lower levels, security and social inclusion, produce each other. A second issue is that notions of human flourishing, or 'eudaimonia' as Aristotle called it, reflect the histories of different individuals, different selves, and different cultures. Aristotle wrote that 'while the good of an individual is a desirable thing, what is good for people or for cities is a nobler or more godlike thing'.[10] Maslow, by contrast, placed self-actualisation at the highest level in his hierarchy. He was writing in 1940s America, at a particular point in the cultural history of Western individualism.[11] Buddhist, Hindu, Confucian and Daoist values might produce other priorities.

Medicine has extended the biological priorities of the emergency-room to most medical encounters, with the result that non-physical needs are constantly being assigned to some other time (after the illness) and to some other place (not the consulting room). The biopsychosocial view of illness[12] nods towards a less hierarchical approach but its role is to clarify the causes of illness rather than to radically disturb medicine's priorities. In both medical education and clinical practice 'getting better' is seen more in physical than in personal terms, despite a theoretical recognition of what are somewhat carelessly dubbed psychosocial factors.

If I am ill, I may not see any problem with deferring the quest for personal well-being. I may imagine that recovery will occur naturally provided a surgeon or a physician or a psychiatrist or a therapist sets me free from the restrictions of illness. Surely I can actualise myself once I am independent? Independence is an important strand in the standard picture of well-being, and was the disability movement's original focus. Neoliberal politics uses the rhetoric of independence because dependency costs money, and the ideal of independence permeates modern health policy[13]. Mutual dependency is, nonetheless, a fact of human life. We are 'patients', as the theologian WH Vanstone says, not solely in illness but also in old age, in retirement, in unemployment and in many other life situations[14]. We are all patients who need someone to collect the refuse and supply drinking water. Vanstone wants us to question whether being looked after is an inherently demeaning position.

> *Denis was a man with disabling MS. He had resolved to end his life because the effects of MS had made him so dependent on other people and on technology. We offered him equipment to compensate for his unsteady arms and paralysed legs, but he rejected all our suggestions.*

I often met people with impairments so severe that they were physically dependent on carers and technologies but who, unlike Denis, seemed able to be themselves. They were intuitively aware of a distinction between independence and autonomy. Autonomy, or 'self-rule', is one of the three keystones in self-determination theory (SDT), a more evidence-based motivation framework than Maslow's.[15] Most of us are autonomous rulers of many aspects of our lives precisely because we can depend on human and technological assistance. I wonder if, for Denis, autonomy was hardly worth having if it consisted solely in passing instructions to a machine that would then deliver food to his mouth. Perhaps he needed also to have the sense of direct physical control over a knife and a fork that only his own limbs could give him. This would be an aspect of mastery, or competence, which according to SDT is another primary motive. In *Someone I used to know* Wendy Mitchell describes dementia slowly taking away her feelings of competence.[16] 'Nothing fazed you' says her new self to her old one, ruefully. Her old self was very competent, loved 'the hustle and bustle of a busy city', and 'always wanted to be busy'. I frequently worked with survivors of brain or spinal cord injuries. These people, mostly young men, were probably often longing, consciously or otherwise, for a return of the sense of preternatural competence that had led them to do dangerous things.

According to SDT, autonomy and mastery/competence sit alongside a third factor, relatedness, which Maslow also emphasizes. What emerges from these motivational theories is the picture of an ideal person whose basic necessities have been met, who has the right amounts of security, self-actualisation, autonomy, competence and self-esteem, and who relates to other people in an ideal way. These are objective attributes, for each of which there are population-based norms. In terms of the WHO's disability frameworks (see p. 26 – Chapter 3) there would be no problems in such a healthy person's 'functioning'. Mental illness has been defined as 'harmful dysfunction'[17] but any form of illness could disrupt biological, psychological and social functioning in basically similar ways.

A standard template of needs gives us a picture of wellness, but pictures have limitations. One problem with both the Maslow and the SDT versions is that they are normative and thus insensitive to what I see as the quintessentially individual nature of ill-being. Their strength lies in their objectivity, which is also their weakness since the needs that ill-being produces arise from within as well as from outside the individual. Generic ideas about wellness are always culturally situated and sometimes absurdly wide of the mark, as we can see in Max Beerbohm's dazzlingly physical and thoroughly gendered caricature of someone who is 'a picture of health':

> He looked, as he himself would undoubtedly have said, 'fit as a fiddle', or 'right as rain'. His cheeks were rosy, his eyes sparkling. He had his arms akimbo, and his feet planted wide apart. His grey bowler rested on the back of his head, to display a sleek coating of hair plastered down over his brow.[18]

Not a captivating picture; and not one that shows the way from ill-being to well-being.

Personal needs

Need, according to a definition used in public health, is the ability to benefit from something that is available.[19] A cure for motor neuron disease can be hoped for, but it is not available at present and so does not count as a person's need from a public health point of view. Someone with pneumonia has a need, and an ability to benefit from, antibiotics. Doctors often describe a treatment as a need, assuming that the patient will benefit without taking the necessary step of enquiring about the person's own desires.

An entirely different definition is implied by describing someone as 'needy'. Need in this sense is a conscious or unconscious yearning that might or might not be beneficial. There is sometimes a contradiction between what we think we can see of a person's needs and what that individual tells us she desires. This might have been true, for example, of Elaine's blindness and Wahid's paraplegia (in Chapter 5), if their symptoms represented some unspeakable dilemma, but on the other hand their symptoms could have met a need that could not be fulfilled in any other way. Ali, with her anorexia (p. 68), had an 'ability to benefit' from food but also had an inner need that nothing could satisfy.

Someone with a mental illness such as psychosis is likely to have an ability to benefit without having the desire to be helped. Defining needs on behalf of someone is ethically perilous. I have an image of Faqar, a man with Huntington's, unable to speak, somewhat emaciated because swallowing was difficult and because constant involuntary movements were burning so many calories. His wife, standing loyally at his bedside, was used to all this but had hardly more certainty than I did about Faqar's state of mind. He was very much alive and alert, but what was he communicating? Was he ill? Most positive possibilities were beyond his own reach. I say most, not all possibilities, because my intuition was that Faqar had some inner competence that still enabled him to control some aspect of his existence. I had felt I had to respond in some way.

Personal needs are difficult to determine because individuals orient themselves towards illness and wellness in very different ways. Each person's responses can be traced, I think, to a self's unique back-story. Three people with motor neuron disease (MND) illustrate some possibilities. First Yvonne, who seemed to me to have found a way of 'coping' with MND. MND plainly brought her grief and fear, but there was something substantial and coherent about her as a person. This was no more than an intuition – what can I know about someone's inner life? – but it was based on observing and experiencing Yvonne in relation to me and also in relation to her husband. Secondly, Eva. I was never on comfortable first-name terms with her. She had withdrawn from everyone, including her husband. Not long after she was diagnosed with MND Eva turned her face literally to the wall: I can picture her now curled up on the sofa, her back towards me, barely uttering a syllable. Something in Eva's self had collapsed. Thirdly, Alan, the most severely disabled of the three, who was living in his elderly mother's house. He was constantly angry with his mother and still had just enough strength in his right leg to kick her. I suspected that these diverse reactions to the same disease reflected the histories of three very different selves.

A person in search of wellness is guided by an aesthetic sense of how things should feel in order for a life to be experienced as one's own. Our desires and fears produce in us needs that diverge from what we are supposed to want, or how we are supposed to behave in illness. The terrain we find ourselves in never has the standard form we are led to expect. Years ago, the film *Love Story* gave me a somewhat romantic picture of leukaemia. I used to imagine that I would display tremendous heroism if I ever got cancer. I probably assumed my sufferings would have a Hollywood soundtrack. Later, when a skin lesion looked to me like a malignant melanoma, I panicked, and lost any chance of being a hero. John Diamond's real experience of cancer collided with a fantasy of himself having a 'close brush', 'a sort of "Death of Chatterton" except that Chatterton gets up off the chaise-longue to write about it'.[20] Illness is nastier and stranger than we can imagine in advance, and what we will desire when we are ill can hardly be predicted. Illness is a strangely unique experience, even if it is a normal one. The same can be said of pregnancy, as Chitra Ramaswamy shows[21], and also of milestones such as puberty, falling in love, ageing, bereavement and death.

Desires

I suggested in Chapter 4 (p. 36) that symptoms produce feelings of burden and also of restriction. These can be translated into practical needs such as safety, in Maslow's hierarchy, or autonomy in SDT. At the same time, they disrupt personal being in less objectifiable ways. 'I am sick, I must die!'; 'I am utterly spent and crushed!'; 'Woe is me!'. These are the cries of a suffering self. They express a longing to be relieved, to be made whole. General theories of wellness cannot accommodate this personal dimension of ill-being. The needs or yearnings that ill-being produces can also be called desires. The distinction I want to make here is not between needs and wants but between needs as objectively defined criteria and needs that are identified uniquely with a particular person and that are that individual's conscious or unconscious desires.

Just as the locus for suffering is a self, so also is the locus for desire. There are objective needs but there are no objective desires. Ali's idea of wellness was a life-threateningly low body weight. Her mother used every argument she could think of to persuade Ali to eat more, to no avail. It was as if we were disputing that yellow was Ali's favourite colour or Ed Sheeran her favourite singer. Ali's notion of wellness was an inner disposition, a feeling, a preference. It was a 'belief' in the warm sense I described in the last chapter (pp. 57–58) – closer to the German belieben, meaning 'like', than to the intellectualized connotations of our word belief. With Ali there was a tension between what she objectively needed, which was food, and what she desired. Here was an especially poignant demonstration of the Buddhist insight that desires are the root of suffering.

Differences between one person's image of wellness and another's often show up in clinical work, although usually producing less dramatic dilemmas than Ali's.

> Gwen (from the last chapter – p. 59) had abandoned her successful career as a businesswoman and was no longer the energetic parent she had formerly been. She insisted that despite her wretched physical symptoms there was something positive about what was happening to her now. She felt closer to her husband James and to her children and granddaughter. Whilst she was proud of what she had achieved she was surprised how little she missed her previous life. As I got to know Gwen she began to describe her early life with a brilliant elder brother, a disabled younger sister and two ambitious but preoccupied parents. She said that since she had been ill she had felt less pressured to please other people.

It seemed to me possible that for Gwen, an outer narrative of success through hard work was in tension with a self-narrative that was more problematic. Yes, she wanted to be productive and useful and she valued the social identity that her career had supported, but she also wanted − desired - something that her illness paradoxically provided.

The seat of desire is the self, but I am far from suggesting that the self is free to desire whatever it likes. Ali was a child, with a limited view of the world. Moreover, she was a child of her time, and hence liable to share the desires of girls like her. Prevalent assumptions about the ideal body were one reason why she felt the need to fast. Gwen's disposition towards illness and wellness depended on her particular perspective, as do everyone's. It takes sociological imagination to see the social origins of one's aspirations, and it takes a different kind of imagination to see how the self's story creates other desires.[22]

Narratives can be traced to two selves that the psychoanalyst Donald Winnicott identifies as the personal private self and the polite or socialised self.[23] The sense that 'I am not myself' belongs more to the private than to the socialised self. The private self's story begins at or perhaps even before birth, from which time an anonymous-seeming neonate gradually becomes an individual in relation to parents and others. Published illness narratives rarely document this intimate narrative, focusing instead on the concerns of a polite and socialised version of the self.[24] A more inwardly-directed story emerges in private conversations and unpublished journals, in psychotherapy, and sometimes in less verbal forms such as dreams and play. Hospitals' efforts to protect 'privacy and dignity' are an attempt (often feeble) to assert the uniqueness of the polite or socialised self, while sometimes entirely disregarding its personal and private counterpart.[25]

The inner self's most basic needs are firstly to exist and secondly to act - to be, and to do. The evidence of psychotherapy suggests that the self's inner story describes a lifelong struggle to 'be'. A fundamental desire in illness is to protect the self's uniqueness, oneness, and continuity. An ill person longs for Laing's ontological security (pp. 39–40). These are attributes that we hardly know we lack until they return to us as we recover from an illness.

One of the expressions of ontological insecurity is, I think, the desire to retreat into a place we can call home, although a person might be longing not so much for a particular house as for the notional space that Bachelard says is 'endowed in our intimate day-dreaming with virtues that have no objective foundation' and that is 'a veritable principle of psychological integration'.[26] Almost no-one feels at home in hospital. Many of our hospitalised patients seemed to imagine that their physical and mental impediments would somehow float away once they were back in their own houses. Who has not had a similar desire to retreat to a private and familiar space in a time of crisis?

The challenges that illness poses for 'doing' are more obvious than those of 'being'. The shrinking and binding effects of illness always reduce one's agency in some degree but as the example of Denis (above) suggests, it is doubtful whether the concept of autonomy fully captures what the self most desires when the will is subverted.

Madeleine, a woman diagnosed with CFS/ME, constantly describes the frustrating contrast between a burning sense of motivation and a body weighed down by heavy legs and overwhelming fatigue: the spirit is willing but the flesh is weak, she says. She sees wellness as the repairing of an engine whose driver, her self, is raring to go.

In depression the self is split at the same somato-psychic border as Madeleine's, but in an opposite way, as though it is the spirit rather than the flesh that is weakened, so that nothing seems worth willing. Wellness would be a rekindling of appetite, desire, participation.

A woman I shall call Sarah revealed more of her self-story than I usually learned.

Sarah had outbursts of aggression towards anyone who tried to help her many mental and physical difficulties. Weakened by a stroke, she would lie semi-supine, almost engulfed in clutter, with books and pictures of religious icons lining the bedroom walls. Her physical environment gave me an image of a crowded, meaning-laden mental landscape. I could make out the shadows of traumas and losses stretching back at least to the time when she was adopted by parents who, she told me, wanted her as a replacement for their dead son. Apparently, Sarah's adoptive father told her he would have preferred a boy. She toyed with the idea that she had multiple selves.

I think that Sarah's mental and also her physical symptoms were damaging the self's unity, coherence and autonomy. These injuries would have to be understood if Sarah was ever to achieve what she herself could call either physical or mental wellness.

Moral resolution

Since the self is where we imagine our actions start, it is also the place where the buck stops. When illness has moral meanings for the sufferer, as described earlier (pp. 67–68), symptoms can be experienced as a very intimate attack on the self. A young woman who came to see us with her twin sister said that she expected to be ill because she was 'the bad twin'. Arthur Frank quotes someone's feeling that she was 'finally being punished' by her illness and was 'paying the price for being a bad mother'.[27] In such circumstances my instinctive response has often been an effort to rescue the damaged self by offering some form of forgiveness. I might imagine that an illusion of guilt has been imposed on the person by sociological pressures, as when blame is first passed into a family by the Big Other of social convention, and then traded from one person to another. Family therapy's success often depends on eradicating blame.[28] Someone is in the grip of an illusion, I often feel, when weighed down with self-blame.

Daphne, (p. 57), insisted that her problems were God's vengeance on her. I felt as if I should challenge Daphne's version of events, which would have involved contesting her worldview. My intuitions might have been well-intentioned, but forgiveness is not in the gift of a doctor or a therapist or anyone else outside a person's moral world, whether an offence has been committed or not. My own culture is suffused with Anglo-American individualism, filtered through a particular, protestant Christian tradition. My thinking has been dominated by the picture of a self in tension with society. As a result, I have been liable to assume that moral well-being depends on somehow enabling a person to stand up for herself against her accusers. Other cultures have a more relational concept of the self, for example Te Ao Māori, the Māori world-view in which interdependence is central, and Zulu ubuntu, in which virtue resides in relationships rather than in individuals, so that well-being is a social state that is closer to Aristotle's eudaimonia than to American-style self-actualisation.[29] In a communal world, blame and guilt must be resolved from within that universe.

When I imagine a tension between a self and a believed-in God, I think of the person standing trial before a detached figure, forgetting that there are people who see good living as an intimate relationship between self, community and God. This is the Hebrew concept of shalom as a wholeness of a person through and in a community rather than in solitude.[30] Someone outside a moral system such as this cannot resolve an injury to it. One therapeutic possibility is to encourage the individual to make a new relationship with her own beliefs. I followed James Griffith's suggestion and asked Daphne if she imagined that her God would want her to suffer, and she said no.[31] Moira (p. 68) had blamed herself for her daughter's illness but a moment later she said 'I agree with my sister. I blame God'. However, she showed me that she had her own ways of adjusting her relationships when she went out of the room saying 'I'll make it up with him [God] when I sweep out the church on Saturday'.

Formal religions create deontological worldviews (from deon, Greek for 'that which is binding, needful, right, proper'). Religious deontology extends beyond ethics to a whole view of how the universe ought to be.[32] A deontological outlook also spreads far beyond organised religions. From a social point of view one can see how cultures make arbitrary evaluations of 'purity and danger' ('eating horses? 'It just isn't right . . . '), but suffering provokes a sense of wrongness that is surely more general. It connects with the sense of natural normality that I discussed in Chapter 3. Anyone who protests that 'no-one ought to die at that age' or that 'she's had more bad luck than anyone ought to have' or even that 'I've had more good luck than I have a right to expect' probably has a culturally inherited vision of moral well-being as a state of nature. Meditating on his own prostate cancer, Anatole Broyard suggests that a 'if the patient can feel that he has earned his illness – that his sickness represents the grand decadence that follows a great flowering – he may look upon the ruin of his body as tourists look upon the great ruins of antiquity'.[33] People seem often to desire some moral dilemma to be resolved in order to feel well. Or to put it the other way round, when one's sense of how the world ought to be is shattered by illness, a coherent vision of the world somehow needs to be repaired or reconstructed as part of the healing process.

Directions

Illness narratives go in different directions – forwards, backwards, in circles, or sometimes nowhere. The simplest trajectory is a return to the point where things went wrong. Arthur Frank calls this a restitution narrative.[34] The restitution route not only looks for a cure but also tries to make the whole of life what it was before, so that one can reappear in one's life at home and at work as though nothing had happened. Heraclitus's famous dictum expresses one problem with the backward path. 'No man ever steps into the same river twice, for it's not the same river, and he's not the same man'. It will be difficult for you to return to status quo after even a short illness because life goes on without you and your position as a patient has made you into a slightly different person. The original river and the original man (or woman) become more and more difficult to recover as illness continues. This is obviously true in chronic illness, especially when changes are simultaneously taking place for other reasons, as in childhood and old age.

> *Adèle, a girl of 13, was brought to us by her mother Bronwen, who told me her daughter was no longer the girl she used to be. For the past five years Bronwen had consulted doctor after doctor about Adèle's mysterious and fluctuating symptoms. She was angered by my attempts to understand the psychological and context of her daughter's illness. 'If you can't cure her I'll take her somewhere else'.*

What Bronwen had in mind was an 8-year-old child who could never have been returned to her, well or ill.

It was not difficult to understand why some of my MS patients made strenuous efforts to force themselves upstream as the disease produced more and more neurological and cognitive impairments. They would seize on whatever miracle cures were currently being touted in the media (gluten-free diets, bee-sting therapy, high-pressure oxygen, vascular treatment) in the sadly mistaken belief that their impairments and disabilities and symptoms could be taken away. A form of nerve damage called demyelination causes the symptoms and impairments of MS, and no technology is yet able to make a person's damaged neurons as good as new. Even if one existed, stepping back into the pre-illness river would still be a challenge. The demand for 'normality' can be unproductive and demoralising but it is often all-absorbing.

Another possible movement in the face of illness is to hide from public view. The shame that stigma produces is one motive. I remember a man with MS who could never be happy until he and his wife were out of town, holed up in their caravan, because in the street where they lived there was so much hostility (he believed) towards disabled people. In the kingdom of the well we can melt into the crowd, but this is not possible while we carry the stigma of illness. As Talcott Parsons said, illness 'isolates and insulates'.[35]

If a ship went back to its home port when blown off course it would produce a restitution narrative. Plotting a new forward course instead of returning home would create what Arthur Frank identifies as a quest narrative.[36] The writer of a published illness narrative is often the protagonist of a sort of Pilgrim's Progress, encountering hobgoblins and foul fiends all over the terrain: some spring from the body; some arise in social relationships; others are personal demons. The challenge is to achieve a hoped-for Good. The quest can be for a personal understanding of illness, for a life beyond suffering, or simply for a different way of enduring life as it is. In *Skybound*, Rebecca Loncraine beautifully describes how she is drawn towards gliding and 'the rapture of flight' in response to a fatal illness. She wants to face fear: 'to choose it, move towards it, become intimate with it' and hence 'to find some freedom from it'.[37]

A quest's holy grail is sometimes moral justification. Any illness can betoken personal weakness, especially in a cultural climate where maintaining one's health is viewed as a duty. The mother who told me she 'doesn't do illness' seemed to be on a permanent quest to demonstrate her moral fibre. A more sympathetic version of the same attitude came from a woman who cheerfully said: 'MS? I'm better than that!'. The quest is often for recognition or validation of an identity. In CFS/ME and other invisible illnesses, including those diagnosed as psychiatric, a person is sometimes forced to resist 'a systematic disconfirmation of the experience of being ill'.[38] In such a climate, the quest may be for the reality of an illness to be recognised and hence for an individual's identity as 'patient' to be validated.

In its simplest form, the quest is for physical recovery and independence, which creates a rehabilitation narrative. The language of goals and outcomes and journeys produces an idealised picture, however. Not everyone wants to take the advice of pop psychology to 'move on', and not everyone is easily motivated by goals. I always taught students that a person without goals could not engage in what we called rehabilitation, but perhaps I was being too strongly influenced by the culture in which I was working. Doctors, nurses and therapists jump through a series of hoops as their careers progress, and healthcare systems are dominated by a culture of targets and outcomes. Some of our patients, I would say the majority, took a very different approach to their illnesses. They preferred to discover what they wanted as they went along rather than specifying the purposes of rehabilitation in advance. A social worker colleague and I hit on a word to describe their to-and-fro movements: they meandered. A meandering course might correspond to Frank's description of a chaos narrative with its seemingly disconnected episodes of 'and then . . . and then . . . ',[39] but meandering need not be as aimless or as chaotic as it seems. In reflecting on what he experienced and observed in concentration camps, Viktor Frankl makes a compelling case for the importance of forward-directed goals as a source of meaning and as a means of survival in times of severe stress.[40] However, he also recognized that at such times the future may be five minutes away (can I make it to the hut?) rather than any larger vision. Many of us feel our way across the contours and struggles of ordinary life, with enough of a sense of the future to give life meaning, but without a clear idea of what life will be like in a year's time. Meandering can be motivated by a kind of hope which, as Kaethe Weingarten says, 'thrives in advance of a coherent image of the future'.[41] Trials and errors are inevitable, and there are countless wrong turnings in any truthful autobiography.

Narratives of strenuous biographical repair over-represent the lives of econom-ically relatively privileged and middle-aged people, because they are the ones with career trajectories.[42] A less celebrated kind of heroism is displayed by those who are determined to stay put and simply 'cope' with chronic and progressive illness. Diane was a woman with significant MS-related disabilities, poor housing and severe family stresses. Her oft-repeated motto, perhaps historically connected with coal-mining, was 'spit on your hands and get on with it'. She would have deemed her life ordinary, and so in one sense it was. Ordinary life rarely has the shape or 'point' of a narrative, and yet the effort required to live her ordinariness took an immense toll on Diane: it was hard to 'be herself'.

> *Pat, a woman with Parkinson's disease, aspired simply 'to be a wife, and to be . . . attractive'. Her husband Don felt that they had 'accomplished things' although 'nothing exceptional'. With their friends they could be happy, but back home they needed to 'let the crap out'.*

This couple were working hard to be themselves both inside and outside their home.

A useful question to ask people with chronic illness is what they would have missed if they had never been ill. The couples I spoke to often felt that they had been brought closer together, and individuals sometimes described being intro-duced through illness to previously unimagined possibilities. A woman in one research study said that 'I think I'm a different person for having come through it, I think it (CFS/ME) has made me a lot stronger than I was, made me face up to things'. A man said that before 'everything was rush rush rush, busy busy busy . . . The illness has made me stop, pause, think, review'.[43] Gwen discovered that inactivity relieved her of some of the pressures of her previous life.

Narratives lend themselves to the externalised view I described in the last chapter (p. 68), making illness something to be 'lived with', as the title of many books about specific diagnoses suggest.[44] Few people want to be entirely identified with a long-term condition such as diabetes or depression or CFS/ME, but ill-being is a form of life that lacks definite boundaries. You would hardly describe yourself as living 'with' flu: for a few days flu is your life, and in a much more radical and permanent way the same is often true in chronic illness. I described earlier (p. 67) how the involuntary movements of Huntington's disease can be appropriated as forms of self-expression. Aspects of many physical and mental illnesses can become almost literally incorporated into the self. To the extent that this has happened it becomes impossible to speak of 'my illness' as something separate.

Self-transformations cannot be narrated by an individual as though they were external events; someone else must witness them. When I was with survivors of severe head injury I often seemed to be watching a movement in the direction of a reconstructed self, a process that had to 'make do' with whatever cognitive and emotional resources happened to be available; twitches that looked like reflex, meaningless responses at one point in time imperceptibly turned into gestures or strategies at another. These were not the movements of an inviolate, disembodied soul or of a body that was merely the slave of biological recovery. They were signs that a person was re-emerging – or so it seemed to me. Elizabeth Fürst gives a moving and academically nuanced description of this process as her own husband recovered from anoxic brain damage.[45]

As a coda to this review of the directions people take in illness, I should finally include the movements that a person makes when terminally ill, in relation to death. At the end of life I have seen many of the patterns already described, such as a desperate effort to reverse an inevitable decline, or a numb stasis, or a ferocious determination to 'rage, rage against the dying of the light', but there are also those who seek out their endings purposefully ('Never weather-beaten sail more willing bent for shore…'). On first noticing blood on his pillow, John Keats is reported to have said: 'that drop of blood is my death-warrant – I must die'. A year after this fateful sign of the consumption that would kill him, he was writing 'Where are the songs of Spring? Ay, where are they? | Think not of them, thou hast thy music too,— While barred clouds bloom the soft-dying day . . .'.[46] Keats' final years were not life-denying, and the same could be said of many of the people I encountered as they negotiated their way through progressive illnesses.

I have been suggesting that part of ill-being's essence is a primal sense of need, which is what binds together an otherwise diverse range of experiences. This chapter reviewed the images of wellness that needs and desires suggest. The final three chapters concern what helps and what gets in the way of positive possibilities.

Notes

1 Winnicott 2016
2 Deegan 1996; see also Field & Reed 2016; Farkas 2007
3 See Hurwitz & Bates 2016; Frank 1997; Kleinman 1988; Bury 1982
4 Lewis 2010
5 Meier et al. 2016
6 WHO 1948
7 Canguilhem 1991, p. 91, quoting Leriche
8 The WHO is defining of pole of a spectrum, for public health purposes
9 Maslow 1987
10 Aristotle, Ed Crisp 2000, Book 1 Chapter 2 1094b
11 Siedentop 2015
12 Engel 1977
13 For example NICE 2013
14 Vanstone 1982
15 Ryan & Deci 2018
16 Mitchell, W. 2017
17 Wakefield 2007.
18 Beerbohm 1923
19 Acheson 1978
20 Diamond 1998, p. 25
21 Ramaswamy 2016
22 Buddhist ideas about desire and the self will take these thoughts in a different direction

23 Winnicott 1990 p. 66: 'each person has a polite or socialised self, and also a private self that is not available except in intimacy . . . [I]n health this splitting of the self is an achievement of personal growth; in illness the split is a matter of a schism in the mind that can go to any depth; at its deepest it is labelled schizophrenia'
24 See Chapter 4. Arthur Kleinman's *Illness Narratives* (1988) is mainly concerned with narrative 'plots' in which illness as an entity causes personal and social repercussions
25 Hospital policies focus on 'basic' or 'inherent' dignity without fully appreciating the personal or aesthetic dimension of dignity – see Pullman 2002 for this distinction
26 Bachelard 1994 p. xxii
27 Frank 1997, p 42
28 Boszormenyi-Nagy & Krasner 1986
29 On ubuntu see Joseph 2018; Tutu 2011, p. 21–24, 172; Masolo 2010, p. 268 (note) and Chapter 4; on Māori worldview see Elder 2015
30 I am grateful to Roy McCloughry for this point. For a view on how Jewish religion produces different notions of communal living see Fishman 2002, pages 5–6 and passim. For a Jewish account of shalom see Shabbat Shalom Magazine 3/11/15. For a Christian perspective see Wolterstorff 1983; Plantinga 1995, p.10: 'The webbing together of God, humans, and all creation in justice, fulfilment, and delight is what the Hebrew prophets call "shalom" . . . a rich state of affairs in which natural needs are satisfied and natural gifts fruitfully employed'
31 Griffith 2010, Chapter 3
32 Plantinga 1995
33 Broyard 1992 p. 48
34 Frank 1997
35 Parsons 1964, Chapter 7
36 Frank 1997
37 Loncraine 2018
38 Ware 1999; see also Cromby 2015b
39 Frank 1997
40 Frankl 1964. I say more about this in Chapter 10
41 Weingarten 2010
42 Williams 2000
43 Whitehead 2006
44 For examples related to MS see: Healthline, https://bit.ly/2J2iOwh

45 Fürst 2015
46 Dylan Thomas "Do not go gentle into that good night'; 'Never weather.'; Thomas Campion 1619; Brown 1841/1937, Life of Keats; John Keats: Ode to Autumn

8

OBSTRUCTIONS

As a doctor I sometimes had the impression that someone was suffering needlessly, as though unwilling or unable to recover any form of well-being. This chapter explores factors that bind us to the terrain of illness. There are obvious biological limitations on the potential to escape illness. In addition, personal difficulties can make wellness unthinkable. Social constraints also get in the way of recovery.

Before considering obstacles to recovery perhaps I should emphasise, as I did in the last chapter, the very broad sense in which I am thinking of recovery. Recovery is to be understood throughout the book as a movement, however slight, in the direction of living well or dying well.

External barriers

The social model of disability has shown that many barriers to well-being are located in society rather than with the impaired individual.[1] A classic example of an environmental obstacle is the steps that prevent a wheelchair user from entering a building. Environmental factors influence the impact of symptoms: fatigue is less of a problem if there is somewhere to rest and if there are people around who understand the need for rest; pain, breathlessness, anxiety and many other symptoms are less restrictive if the right social attitudes, practices and policies are in place. On the other hand, it is clearly possible to exaggerate the extent to which well-being can be produced by environmental changes and social policies even when funds are unlimited. This is better recognised in the recent than in the older disability literature: Tom Shakespeare writes that 'even after discrimination and prejudice is removed, inequalities are likely to remain. The level playing field does not liberate everyone'.[2] Just as there may be no way of removing some of the burdens that chronic pains or shortness of breath produce, so there may be no possibility of relief from impairments that disease causes. Each body has certain capacities and certain limitations that cannot be modified; this is as true in health as it is in disease. Moreover, a person's conceptions of well-being often go beyond what is physically possible. The nature of Denis's impairments (p. 76) meant that equipment could not compensate for his sense of physical incompetence.

Positive psychology is reluctant to admit the power of physical facts to stand in the way of well-being, but no amount of positive thinking alters the way chronic pain attenuates the inner life, and many psychiatric symptoms are equally resistant to positive strategies.[3] Anyone close to a person with severe depression will encounter a leaden resistance in that person's entire being, something that has an almost bodily feel to it. The black dog can defeat even the strongest of spirits, just as cancer can. It somehow blocks the path towards wellness.

It is also tragically true that from the perspective of someone who is ill there are certain social conditions that have the status of physical facts even though they are the effects of political and economic power and could potentially be removed. Many industries cause or exacerbate specific diseases. A man on one of our medical wards was dying a terrible death from respiratory failure due to asbestosis. He remembered having snowball fights with handfuls of asbestos whilst renovating a power station in the 1960s, despite the fact that the dangers of asbestosis had first been noted before World War I. His fate had been sealed by forces that were controllable, but not by him. Some of the social stresses that aggravate anxiety and place limits on a person's ability to recover either personally or socially are produced by factors that socio-logical imagination would reveal, and that political action could change, but from the individual's point of view they are an unmovable barrier to well-being.

Inner blockages

Indifference

One of the most disabling effects of illness is to take away desire, making a person indifferent to her fate. Patricia Deegan describes her 17-year-old self, undergoing medical management of her psychotic illness: 'People come and people go. People urge her to do things to help herself but her heart is hard and she cares about nothing except sleeping, sitting, and smoking cigarettes'.[4] Physical as well as mental illness suppresses one's basic appetites. The torpor that illness produces is different from Denis's coldly rational rejection of help, or from the passionate feelings of Ali (p. 68), who so vigorously resisted everyone's efforts to persuade her to eat. There are times when even death can be a matter of indifference rather than something that is either feared or welcomed. On one of my last ward rounds as a physician I talked to a woman who was lying supine on her hospital bed. I asked her what would happen if she didn't drink enough fluid. She replied with a question: 'Wouldn't I go into a coma?' 'And would you care if you died?' 'Not particularly'. She smiled. This was probably not so much a desire to die as indifference to her fate. The therapeutic interventions we were busying ourselves with were beside the point from this woman's point of view.

People sometimes resist therapeutic efforts because they don't accept that they are ill. In the neurological state called anosognosia a person is unable to perceive, for example, the effects of a stroke. For similar reasons certain forms of amnesia are not apparent to the individual, who confabulates wildly because no gaps in memory are noticed.[5] Other forms of indifference occur in psychiatric conditions and in situations I mentioned in the last chapter (p. 78), where someone makes no claim to feel ill and yet appears to others to be patently unwell. Lack of congruence between the person and others is most familiar to us in psychological denial, as when someone with cancer refuses vital treatment on the grounds that 'it will be alright' (see Chapter 10 for more on denial). Many of these cases, I think, are best thought of as indifference to disease, rather than to illness. One of this book's basic tenets is that the existence or non-existence of illness cannot be contradicted by others. A person might not have the mental capacity to recognise practical needs, for example for cancer treatment, but however deluded a person may be there is always something valid about her claim to have no problems. She might have a disease, but she cannot be experiencing ill-being, as I conceive it, if she denies feeling distressed.

On the other hand, there are surely times when ill-being is visible to others and yet not expressed by the sufferer. This was how I thought of Faqar, the man with Huntington's disease described in the last chapter (p. 78). A very different version of the same dilemma was Lori (p. 58). There was a disturbing incongruity between her dramatic, medically inexplicable symptoms and her look of contentment. Was she ill? She fitted the profile of conversion disorder, and I think she was displaying what nineteenth century French neurologists mockingly called 'la belle indifférence'. If they had taken the trouble to explore this apparent indifference, as Freud soon afterwards did, they might have unearthed personal and relational sufferings that could be called illness. I think Lori was 'not herself', and that something in her was blocking the possibility of wellness.

Doctors and others who suspect that someone is not trying to be well can rapidly become hostile. People who do not co-operate can be seen as 'declining voluntarily and openly to accept the social place accorded them'; by rejecting help they are acting 'irregularly and somewhat rebelliously in connection with our basic institutions'[6] – in this case, the institutions of healthcare and rehabilitation. Such righteous anger towards non-compliant people has the paradoxical effect of still further reducing their chances of taking steps towards recovery, because it increases the need to be seen as ill. When doctors feel over-confident about who is ill and who is well. they are on a slippery slope that begins with diagnostic arrogance about other people's feelings and ends ultimately in flagrant abuses.

Desiring safety

The compensations of illness are a well-known barrier to recovery. The sick role, as Talcott Parsons called it,[7] certainly has advantages, some of which I discussed in Chapter 5 (p. 46; 50). However, I do not think that the sick role is such a strong inducement to remain ill as is commonly imagined. Many people have flimsy excuses for 'calling in sick', but illness as an excuse for a day off does not equate with illness as a way of life. Someone who fabricates illness or who seems to be drawn towards the sick role has to endure stigma, must sacrifice a great deal of autonomy, and inevitably falls under the jurisdiction of doctors and agencies that promote re-employment and minimize costs. There is work involved in pretending to be ill, as I pointed out in Chapter 5. In exchange for all this, the financial benefits of illness are relatively meagre. Evidence is scarce because malingerers are not willing participants in research, but I suspect that most of those who get stuck in the sick role are held there less by the desire to be unemployed or to sponge off the state than by the other factors I am considering here. In the first place, so-called social security benefits are not merely financial. A sick role might provide literal social security to someone who otherwise feels unsure of a place in society.

In my medical work I met many people who seemed unwilling to face the prospect of recovery after a long illness. There were those who clung to a diagnostic label, and those who seemed to be more at home in hospital than back in their normal lives. It is too easy to dismiss such attitudes as selfish, weak or devious. Making the best of where you find yourself is both necessary and natural. Think what it might be like to spend a few months in another country. As time passes you will steadily acquire more of the apparatus you need to survive: bedding, cutlery and so on. At the same time a social existence will be forming. In the Kingdom of the Sick, many people come towards you when you are ill, offering acceptance, friendship, and assistance and perhaps, in return, you become literally or morally indebted to them. What was originally foreign territory has now become a safe haven and moving away from it is a challenge.

> *The pull of illness was obvious for an elderly woman called Millie, who produced countless symptoms whenever the possibility of discharge from hospital was mentioned. She preferred the comfort and camaraderie of a warm four-bedded ward to her solitary existence at home.*
>
> *For teenaged Clio the attraction of hospital was even stronger. She had been admitted because of suicidal depression, which was connected with her fractured family life. Some of the nurses and young patients she met during her stay became her substitute family, offering support she could not get elsewhere. Hospital life relieved her distress, which helps to explain how she came to be readmitted on three further occasions.*

Families living with long-term illness develop a way of life that is vitally significant for them. As a result, two people – sometimes more – may become more mired in the terrain of illness than they need to be.

> *Lena's MS had produced severe disabilities. Her husband devoted his life to caring for her. Lena's physical position, in bed and propped up on pillows, corresponded to her relational position as Tomasz's 'patient'.*

Imagining Lena's point of view, we wondered if Tomasz was in some ways a barrier to her well-being. When someone like Lena died, we often observed how difficult it was for the person's carer to separate from a network of relationships with nurses, social workers and others. For similar reasons, people who are completely cured of cancer sometimes find it hard to leave a place where their suffering has been understood. Such situations remind me of Jamie, in *Empire of the Sun*.[8] When he suddenly found he could leave the concentration camp, he thought twice before walking free. Anyone for whom illness becomes a safe haven is liable to become what David Lodge calls an unhappy hoper.[9] To spare themselves pain, unhappy hopers set their sights low, almost revelling in the failure of therapeutic efforts, and steering clear of uncertainty.

Several of the last chapter's stories suggest that experiences in earlier life can limit a person's ability to accept help in times of distress. Sarah's turbulent relationships with doctors, therapists, carers and friends very probably derived from her adoptive parents' difficulty in supplying sufficient care in early life. The anger of the two people with motor neurone disease, Eva and Alan, perhaps had similar sources. The gain that people are assumed to be seeking when they feign illness or get stuck in the sick role is sometimes the possibility of being cared for in a more positive way than they have experienced as developing selves. The 'needy' person often is someone whose needs never have been met.

Obstructive relationships

Politics is about power. Politics is everywhere because, as Michel Foucault said, 'power is everywhere'.[10] According to one definition, power is 'a determining force that causes some people to get less and some more of whatever is considered desirable in a social world'.[11] This makes power sound like a tankful of fuel or a stash of Kalashnikovs, but it is better to think of it as a product of relationships. The power differentials between family members, or between doctors and patients, or between nations, are all built on relationship patterns that in some circumstances create or perpetuate illness.

Personal relationships

The systemic concept of positioning gives an account of the way relationships at all levels trap people in the sick role. Positioning occurs between two or more people who adopt complementary relationships with one another. One can be positioned within a family or any small or large group as disabled or able bodied; genuinely ill or fake; deserving or undeserving; and so on. Harré and colleagues describe positioning in terms of meanings, expressed in cognitive terms and focusing especially on the rights and duties that play out in 'story-lines'.[12] Rights and duties here are 'shorthand terms for a cluster of moral (normative) presuppositions which people believe or are told or slip into and to which they are momentarily bound in what they say or do'.[13] 'Momentarily' is important here. Unlike roles, positions can be created instantaneously, as when Mrs Jones is given the 'seat of honour' in the doctor's consulting room, with the duty to describe her symptoms and the right to be heard. The doctor shows Mr Jones to a subsidiary place in the room, where he may be positioned as carer by being asked to help his wife remove her shoes. The opposite seating arrangement, often seen when the patient is assumed to be cognitively impaired, positions Mr Jones as spokesman, with Mrs Jones positioned as a mute, helpless object of clinical interventions. With the chairs side by side, a different narrative may be discovered. In the position of patient, a person has the right to be cared for but also a duty to try to get well.[14] Someone positioned as carer has clear duties, although few rights, so that these complementary positions involve a redistribution of power.

> *The behaviour of Violet, age 14, has always been disruptive, and her relationships with other family members are stormy. Violet has been diagnosed with autism spectrum disorder (ASD). She has been positioned in her family as 'the girl with autism'. In the family's narrative, autism is an illness, even though Violet does not feel or look ill. Her parents no longer blame Violet for the problems she causes but by the same token she has less responsibilities. Her parents fear that tasks such as emptying the dishwasher will exacerbate Violet's symptoms, so her brother is left with this job.*

Violet has gained the rights – the powers – that attach to a sick person, and by implication everyone else in the family is positioned as her carer. So small an act as to declare autism to be a difference rather than a deficit, a source of disability rather than an illness, will lead to a new pattern of positions that may have liberating effects for all concerned.

People with long-term illness or disability are frequently positioned as patients who receive care and from whom nothing is expected. An invalid, almost by definition, lacks autonomy. In Henry James' novel *Portrait of a Lady*, Ralph Touchett has consumption. He describes himself as 'ill and disabled and restricted to mere spectatorship at the game of life'.[15] When one member of a couple has been positioned as patient and the other as carer the effects on the relationship can be profound.[16] It is hard to be both a carer and a lover. This was a dilemma for Melanie, whose physical abilities were being steadily eroded by MS, and for her partner Dan. They wanted to escape the patient/carer language that was being forced on them by Melanie's increasing physical dependency. Melanie and Dan discovered ways of resisting the way the world wanted to describe them, and so did a 75-year-old woman named Cheryl, showed that abandoning a position can be a conscious choice.

> *I was asked to see Cheryl on a medical ward. She had a neurological disorder that had been very slowly progressing for many years. Everyone – her family, her GP and hospital staff – described Cheryl as 'fiercely independent'. Nurses and therapists on the ward were therefore puzzled and frustrated when she proved unwilling to help them set her up at home again, following an episode of infection. What she told me, out of the*

staff's hearing, was that she had been watching preparations for other patients to leave the hospital and had noticed them receiving more funding and more home equipment than she had ever had.

Cheryl had decided that she wished to retire from the hard work of looking after herself. She now wanted to adopt a different position, a new role, as someone who is looked after. The pathway towards Cheryl's idea of well-being was being blocked by the way she was being positioned by others.

Gender, and its effects on illness and help-seeking, is another, clearly political manifestation of positioning. The father of Jordan (p. 94), gives us an example of the way society confers power on men: he was in a position not only to leave Jordan's mother, Shelley, with responsibility for Jordan but also to criticise her as a parent. From a sociological perspective Shelley's own ill health prompts us to consider how her trouble might connect with the relative powerlessness of many women, and with the higher prevalence of psychiatric diagnoses in women than in men.

Defending an identity

The position of patient creates an identity, and sometimes the identity of sick person is as difficult to pull off as a hospital wrist-band. I doubt if I would have become a doctor had I not been, at 13, the youngest patient in an adult hospital ward. My experience confirms Juredeini and Taylor's observation that 'illness can be a special experience for the child or its parent'; 'hospitals, being nursed in bed, and medical treatment not only offer attention and caring, but also can create relatively good feelings out of adversity',[17] Many writers on their own illness, for example Porochista Khakpour and Lauren Slater,[18] describe these positive effects. Illness identity might distract a person from turning towards wellness partly because, like a wrist-band, it provides an entrance ticket to the domain where the valuable relationships I have just been describing have formed: with other patients, and with those who have cared for you and about you. Illness identity, especially in the form of a diagnosis, is also difficult to abandon if it provides the key to services, a point I will return to later.

Concerns about identity reduce the chance of being well in an opposite way when shame or fear discourage someone from seeking help. I remember an elderly woman I saw when I was a student. She had come on her own to see a surgeon, complaining of a 'sore place' on her breast. On the examination couch she very reluctantly revealed a cancerous ulcer that she had been harbouring for months. Families with Huntington's disease are just as often reluctant to be identified.

A striking example was James, whose symptoms had been progressing for years, until the time when they were too obvious to ignore. His wife Margaret, who had been devotedly caring for him and holding the family together without help, rejected almost every suggestion we made, preferring to return to the privacy of the family home.

A sense of stigma was separating Margaret, James and the family from resources that we thought could have helped them lead somewhat happier lives.

Stigma also has a way of perpetuating an illness identity by labelling a person as 'damaged goods'. An identity such as 'recovering MS' or 'mental health problem' that has been casually attached to an unwell person can long outlast the illness. If your public identity is stigmatized in these ways, you may yourself come to feel diminished, hopeless and in a sense ill. The label that has been applied to you has what has been called the 'Why try?' effect[19], which holds you in the terrain of illness.

Sometimes the alternative to maintaining an illness identity is to be accused, retrospectively, of malingering. Hypnosis gave Wahid (p. 49) a chance to throw away his crutches without being exposed to the accusation that his illness never had been genuine. If his friends had been raising funds to send him to America for specialist treatment it would probably have been more difficult to abandon the identity of a helpless invalid. Those diagnosed with CFS/ME and other contested labels face a similar dilemma. They must often devote a lot of energy to defending their credibility because they encounter 'systematic disconfirmation'. Illness experience must be confirmed, and a person must be seen to qualify for the sick role. A sense of qualification is often bolstered by fellow-sufferers, through self-help groups, and renouncing one's right to be ill might then be seen as a betrayal of other people as well as of oneself. Illness disqualifies you in many ways: you might no longer qualify for the power or the prestige you once had; you might literally be disqualified from driving. In exchange you qualify for financial benefits, for support, and perhaps for care. Renouncing one's position as ill is to renounce one's qualifications, which takes courage.

Helping systems

Ideally, human services should be organised around people's problems. When a road accident triggers the arrival of an ambulance and a police car, the response usually is needs-led or 'problem-determined'.[20] Modern health services are usually protocol-led rather than problem-determined. The fit between a standard protocol and a standard problem such as a road accident can be close enough for the system to seem to be problem-determined, but the problems that turn up in an emergency room or a GP's surgery rarely have a standard form and illness, as a uniquely personal experience, never does. When the medical machine grinds on without being able to adapt to individual needs it becomes a problem-generating system rather than a problem-determined one.

Medicine has a notorious tendency to make people physically ill through the complications of investigations, drugs, surgery and, above all, hospitalisation. Hospitals contribute physically to the construction of illness by sapping energy, dampening mood and reducing appetite. Being frailer and less confident than before, people recovering from illness are often discouraged from getting back to work and hence become dependent on medical confirmation that they are still unwell. This was a situation I frequently faced when I was asked to certify a patient's fitness for work. Someone's claim to be ill might seem doubtful but I could see nevertheless that re-employment would make that person again unwell. A crude sick/well dichotomy often made it seem necessary for me to err on the side of endorsing illness even when it might have been more accurate to describe a person as well, although still vulnerable.[21]

Financial and other benefits that are directly related to medical assessments have the effect of welding people to their medical identities, especially when the alternative will be poverty and debt. Conversely, the lack of a medical diagnosis undermines a claimant's credibility even with services that profess to assess needs on non-medical criteria. Diagnosis is just as critical in mental as in physical illness. Child and Adolescent Mental Health services (CAMHS) are only available for young people with an established psychiatric diagnosis. Diagnosis unlocks sources of educational support so that undoing the diagnosis and returning to the 'well' category is difficult. These are examples of the paradoxical tendency of helping systems to perpetuate illness identity.

People report their difficulties in whatever terms are appropriate to the services they use:

> *Paul, a man with MS, was bombarding the specialist nurse with phone calls about relatively minor symptoms. When we made an opportunity for Paul and his wife to talk more generally about their experience of MS it became clear to us all that they were very distressed about their own relationship and about their son's difficulties. Paul's physical symptoms faded into the background once the non-medical issues began to be addressed, and calls for medical and nursing help became rare.*

The very existence of our specialist service was having the effect of increasing Paul's preoccupation with the medical aspect of his MS; it was making him 'ill'. Millie, the woman who felt at home in hospital, provides another example of system-determined problems. Hospital admission exacerbated her feelings of loneliness and undermined her sense of competence, not least because the safety-obsessed hospital system would not allow Millie even to go to the toilet independently, let alone cook for herself. The medical setting paradoxically encouraged her to feel ill and to dread whatever ideas of wellness (i.e. independence) the doctors might suggest to her.

Jordan's experience is also an example of a problem-generating system. The school nurse noticed that Jordan was cutting herself. She suspected that Jordan's self-harm was a symptom of her home situation rather than of mental illness but there was no non-medical service available to support the family's distress. The only option was the local CAMHS which interpreted Jordan's difficulties in terms of medical diagnoses. A medical formulation proved to be misleading and probably damaging to this girl and her family. If Jordan had encountered a problem-determined system her mood might have been seen as a response to her environment rather than being labelled as anxiety. Her OCD-like behaviours might have been interpreted as a vulnerable young person's anxious effort to control at least something in her very uncertain world. Diagnostic labels might or might not also have been useful, but both the school and the family doctor would have been geared to the needs of the family as a whole.

The current UK government decrees that mental health services for people like Jordan 'should not be based solely on clinical diagnosis but on the presenting needs of the child or young person'.[22] However, the same government's policies militate against this ideal by reducing social services. Neoliberal economic ideology has the effect of promoting medical diagnostic labelling because in a competitive health market a medical diagnosis supplies a visible 'brand' whereby a 'product' can be defined. This is one among several reasons why services are commissioned specifically for eating disorders, CFS/ME, breast cancer, etc rather than being flexibly responsive to individual needs. Family-oriented work is not seen as the primary business of the health 'industry', because it seems too remote from healthcare's core business.

Jordan's and Paul's stories show how the structure of services can produce a restricting, medical view of human distress. Specialist services, for example CAMHS, can only be accessed if diagnostic criteria are met. I often felt motivated to diagnose CFS/ME since this would enable someone to access our excellent specialist therapies. The use of prescribed medications is another factor that strengthens a person's relationship with illness and with medical systems. Jordan's status as an ill individual was constantly being reaffirmed by her visits to doctors, who were monitoring a drug she was being given for her OCD, just as the drugs prescribed for Paul's symptoms gave him a medical ticket. Investigations have a similar anchoring effect. If you fear being regarded as well you can always ask for another test, just in case. Conversely, it is difficult not to feel and behave like someone who is ill whilst you are awaiting an investigation. These are all aspects of medicalisation.

Macro politics

Sociological imagination is needed to see that some of the most powerful barriers to wellness are the result of decisions that politicians have either made or failed to make. Millie's desire to remain in hospital, for example, reflected the fact that investment in acute medical services had been prioritised over social services, so that hospital was her only chance of receiving the attention she needed. Medicalisation has been encouraged by a politically-motivated shift in the UK towards a market model of healthcare that thrives on diagnoses and specialist services, so that responsibility for many system-determined problems can be laid at the feet of those who hold political power. The individual situations that we tend to analyse in terms of personal motivation and family context are seen in a different light from a sociological point of view. Jordan's medical formulation was constructed and sustained by the power vested in school and health services. The family's poverty was the effect of a social and economic order in which there is a widening divide between winners and losers. The fragmentation of Jordan's family was thus not just a piece of misfortune for these particular people but also a symptom of the oppressive social system in which the family lived. Jordan herself was virtually powerless, although we might wonder if her poor school attendance was an act of resistance and her self-harm an inarticulate protest against her powerlessness.

Few of my patients were interested in making connections between their private troubles and public issues, even if they had a political turn of mind. Mills might have been speaking of Jordan's family when he wrote: 'Is it any wonder that ordinary people feel they cannot cope with the larger worlds with which they are so suddenly confronted? That they cannot understand the meaning of their epoch for their own lives?'[23] Doctors and other healthcare professionals are also ordinary people, equally lacking in sociological imagination. They often describe themselves as apolitical but they operate within systems that have powerful effects and that do have political implications.

Notes

1 Oliver 1996, p. 32
2 Shakespeare 2018
3 See Ehrenreich (2009) for a vigorous critique of positive psychology
4 Deegan 1996
5 As in alcohol-induced Korsakoff's syndrome
6 Goffman 1968, p. 143
7 Parsons 1964, Chapter 7: Deviant Behavior and the Mechanisms of Social Control; see also Chapter 10: Social Structure and the Dynamic Process: The Case of Modern Medical Practice
8 *Empire of the Sun*, novel by JG Ballard, film by Steven Spielberg
9 Lodge 1995
10 Foucault 1978
11 Lemert 2005
12 Hollway 1984
13 Harré et al. 2009
14 Parsons 1964. Chapter 7
15 Henry James 1881. *Portrait of a Lady*. Chapter 15
16 See Ward 2012
17 Jureidini & Taylor 2002; Khakpour (2018); Slater (2000)
18 Khakpour 2018; Slater 2000.
19 Corrigan et al. 2009
20 Harlene Anderson and colleagues developed the idea of a problem-determined system in a somewhat different context (Anderson et al. 1986; Anderson & Goolishian 1988)
21 See note on ambivalence in Chapter 5 (note 25, p.55); see also Ward 2015b
22 Department of Health, 2015
23 Mills 1959, Chapter 1

9

RESOURCES

The last chapter identified hindrances to wellness. This one and the next are about what helps. They are addressed to health workers, including not only nurses, doctors and therapists but also sick persons and their families and friends.[1] My guiding image here, as everywhere in the book, is a sick person. Let's go back to Zola. She is one of the health workers herself, tasked with trying to be better. Better is a relative term rather than a synonym for perfect health, and recovery, as I define it, is a movement towards life rather than an endpoint. Recovery in this sense would be possible for Zola even if she was on her deathbed. Zola is finding it impossible to will wellness and knows she will be saddled with her suffering unless she can find supportive resources.

The most obvious destination for Zola is her doctor, but I will be arguing that her foundational resource is healing, not medical cure. Perhaps a health warning is needed here. I risk scouring so much varnish off medicine's flaky image that there will be nothing left. Modern medicine is hugely helpful, as I well know, but I invite you to think critically about how it helps. The word physician comes from the Greek phusis, nature, and what we call cure is usually best regarded as a collaboration with natural processes rather than a substitute for them.

This chapter's first task will be to consider the meanings of healing, the conditions that promote it, and its relationship to medical interventions. A more mundane resource is money. Money is one form of capital, but there are non-monetary resources that are social capital, and another bankable resource for Zola is reserve capacities that might lessen the impact of injury on her body or mind. Finally, there are personal relationships. Rather than thinking of them as social capital (which in a sense they are), I have in mind the contributions that only persons can make to the healing process. Robots can deliver interventions but only human beings recognise and empathise with suffering. They provide comfort and on occasions consolation, and they accompany a person through the otherwise very solitary experience of illness.

Healing

Medicine, in all its orthodox and non-orthodox forms, supplies a menu of remedies ranging from cough mixture to chemotherapy. The magical ideal is a cure which makes us good as new, able to continue life as though illness had never happened. The list of illnesses that can be cured is woefully short. As medical technology strides ahead, people are more and more surprised by this. When I asked groups of medical students to tell me about some patient they had seen being cured, they were disturbed to realise that almost all hospital work is about chronic and recurrent conditions. GPs have a slightly better time, since ailments such as boils and athlete's foot and allergies can be magicked away with drugs but most medical problems cannot. 'Job done!' my GP said, offering me steroids for a skin condition, but we both knew that the problem was due to a process that was far from done: ageing.

Victorian physicians used to wring their hands with the words 'We can do so little' (the sly ones might say 'If only you'd called me earlier'). Physicians mostly adopted an 'expectant' strategy, implying that the disease would run its natural course before the patient recovered. Today's doctors are often expectant, although instead of hovering helplessly at the bedside, they are likely to busy themselves ordering investigations, or organising non-specific interventions such as intravenous fluids.

Only when the doctor's and the pharmacist's cupboards are bare and every conceivable diagnostic test has been done are we liable to notice that the resource we are in most need of in illness is healing. The word remedy derives from mederi, a Latin word translated as healing, but not even antibiotics heal the body. Their role is to remove bacteria, leaving the inflamed and dysfunctional tissues to heal in some other way. Healing is a word that is often used by doctors and nurses but almost absent from the medical curriculum. Victorian doctors called themselves practitioners of the healing art, but healing barely merited a mention in their textbooks. The index of Sir Clifford Allbutt's monumental eight-volume *System of Medicine* (1899) goes straight from 'Head-nodding' to 'Heart, diseases of'. The equally massive *Oxford Textbook of Medicine* (2010) indexes 'Headache' and then 'Health advertising'.[2]

The French and the Germans seem able to do without a specific word for healing; guérir and heilen respectively cover the English terms healing and also cure. Both guérir and heilen can be used transitively, in phrases such as 'I cured you', and also intransitively, as in 'the wound will heal'. A doctor who says she heals people is very like a gardener who says she grows tomatoes. In both cases the grammar has slipped: healing and growing are not someone's actions; they are processes that are difficult for any of us either to start or to stop.[3]

Not a single drug, at the time of writing, will reliably accelerate the healing of a surgical wound or a fracture. Some of our most useful drugs, such as steroids, actually delay healing. Alternative medicine is equally powerless to heal. There isn't a herb on the planet that can directly bring about healing (if one existed, Monsanto would probably have patented it long ago). Doctors and others create the conditions for healing just as gardeners create the conditions for growth. A surgeon who stitches two edges of a wound together is helping to regulate the natural healing process, just as a gardener helps a plant by providing a trellis. I think of psychotherapy as aligning the raw edges of a psychic wound to make it more possible for some inner process to knit them together successfully.

Another word for healing is recovery. Recovery suggests the same kind of autonomous process as healing. Just as it is you who heals, so it is you who recovers; no-one else can do the job for you.[4] One advantage of the term 'recovery' is its connotations of salvage. A recovering market is saved from collapse when it reaches an equilibrium that economists describe as healthy; and to recover from any illness is to be brought back from a perilously unstable state. The idea of saving is deeply embedded in the language of healing and cure. The Indo-European root of guérir is said to include the idea of defending or protecting; heilen derives from a different stem that also has connotations of saving. One of the words in New Testament Greek that is translated as healing is sozo, which also means save, as when a blind person is able to see because his faith has saved him.[5] Saving ideas often remain close to the idea of wholeness, which is a strand in the meaning of heilen and hence of health and healing.[6] The body-self is 'saved' simultaneously in both a physical and a spiritual sense through a restoration of its original integrity, its wholeness, its 'health'. A surgeon who debrides gangrenous tissue can save a limb that would otherwise have to be amputated, just as someone in a diabetic coma can be saved from biochemical chaos by insulin.

Psychological recovery, or resilience, can be thought of as a person's ability to 'bounce back emotionally from stressful events'.[7] Systems ideas, introduced in Chapter 1, help to make healing and recovery less mysterious. Any system tends to bounce back when it is perturbed. A mechanical system such as a bridge literally bounces when the wind strikes it, and a biological system has a similar tendency to maintain its original conditions when put under stress, which is how it adapts to the vagaries of weather, diet and so on. Skin, for example, is a system of specialised cells that responds to day-to-day stresses such as mechanical forces and changes in temperature. The same system's response to a skin wound is what we call healing.[8] Many systems both within and beyond the brain must somehow recover their function before walking is again possible after a stroke. When a person's existence is torn apart by either a mental disturbance such as depression or a physical one such as stroke, recovery involves innumerable adjustments in the internal and external relationships that make up the body-self's system, its way of being. Recovery is a movement from one state of the system – the 'other life' that I described in Chapter 3 – towards a different state.

There are two ways of describing recovery after an acute illness. Physical healing has a defined time course, but personal recovery can continue indefinitely. We used to tell students that recovery from a stroke was largely complete within three months, which is true from a biological point of view, but a person's new, post-stroke life may still be developing for months or years beyond that point. A woman called Gwyneth was close to the 12-week point when therapists began telling her husband Mick that she would never walk again. She left the ward in a wheelchair. Six months later, Mick brought Gwyneth triumphantly back. They wanted to celebrate the fact that she could now take a few effortful steps. Her walking was not much use from a functional point of view, but she and Mick had worked very hard since leaving hospital to achieve a symbolic goal, which was for Gwyneth to 'get back on her feet'. This was not cure, but it was healing of a kind.

Regimens

Healing is only possible if the conditions are right, a principle that pre-modern medicine expressed in the idea of a therapeutic regimen. A regimen was formed from the six 'non-naturals' of Hippocratic medicine: air; food and drink; excretion; passions and emotions; sleeping and waking; and motion and rest.[9] Rest made intuitive sense – who does not long to be asleep when ill? – and it was often a key element in a patient's regimen. London surgeon John Hilton's book *Rest and Pain* went through six editions between 1863 and 1950, with its case histories of 'abscess – cured by rest. . . . hip-disease in a scrofulous patient – cured by rest . . . '.[10] Rest was often the only possible remedy, and it sometimes worked. Damaged tissues do need dressings or sutures or slings to immobilise them while they heal. Rest was the mainstay of treatment for consumption, as pulmonary tuberculosis was called.[11] The answer to neurasthenia, CFS/ME's Victorian ancestor, was the rest cure according to the American neurologist Weir Mitchell, whose methods became popular on both sides of the Atlantic.[12]

The culinary side of Mitchell's therapeutic regimen consisted of a diet that he summarised, bizarrely, as 'blood and fat'. Ill people were always urged to eat well while they rested (I rather envied Hans Castorp's two breakfasts, taken as part of a consumptive's regimen in *The Magic Mountain*[13]). Foods have often been used as medicines, and still are.[14] Fresh air and sunlight were other elements in the regimen. Florence Nightingale-inspired Victorian hospitals had large windows and balconies reminiscent of the luxurious veranda on which Hans Castorp breathed mountain air.[15] The curative properties of water have an ancient pedigree that was thoroughly medicalised in the nineteenth century. Rest, air, sun, water, food: these were the remedies of Hippocratic medicine. Even though the four humours (Yellow Bile, Black Bile, Phlegm, Blood) and the four elements (Air, Fire, Earth, Water) of Hippocratic doctors have been firmly set aside by orthodox physicians for nearly two centuries, similar ideas survive in modern societies.[16] The science may be shaky but the underlying intuition is sound, that nature is a resource for restoring the balance of health. There are shreds of evidence to confirm the therapeutic effect of a natural environment. In one hospital, the outcomes following a specific operation were statistically slightly better for patients who happened to occupy beds where there was a rural view.[17]

Places

The Greek god Asclepius's shrine at Epidauros was a place of sanctuary, a peaceful locale designed to aid a spiritual healing process (along with medical treatment). Monastic hospitals were places that fostered both kinds of healing through a regimen of care, food, shelter and prayer. The wards in Victorian hospitals, following Florence Nightingale's principles, were not technological workshops. They were supposed to be places of healing that were airy, clean, well-lit and soothing, with patients' spiritual needs typically catered for in a magnificent chapel. Because rest was so important you would be handed over, body and soul, to a regiment of nurses and doctors and chaplains: you would be a patient. Activity would be gently reintroduced as you recovered, ideally in a convalescent home with a rural or seaside setting to rival the Alps.[18] Vast 'lunatic asylums' for people were built on similar lines, with the same assumption that architecture and setting were agents of healing. They were surrounded by gardens where, it was imagined, inmates would recover their senses as they tilled the soil.

There is no place for rest within contemporary medicine. Recovery and healing have been 'dis-placed' by ceaseless activity. Ironically, intensive medicine has recycled the word recovery as a programme of aggressive rescue activities. The recommended therapy for CFS/ME, today's version of neurasthenia, is not rest but graded exercise. In medicine and surgery, exercise is de rigeur, just as rest once was. Exercise combats depression, hypertension and osteoarthritis. Activity improves the outcomes of surgery, with lower mortality, less pain, less infection, less deep venous thrombosis. A day or two after even a major operation you will be urged on to your feet, and in a startlingly short period of time you are likely to be shown the door. Your destination will be your home, not the Alps or even the seaside. Convalescent homes are a thing of the past, but so also is the very notion of convalescence. As a hospital-based rehabilitationist, I constantly preached a gospel of action. We were always hoping to 'get the patient going', with the tacit assumption that unwellness would then fade away of its own accord. It often did, but a person's sense of being ill, of not being herself, was a distraction from our primary mission and not something that we specifically responded to. It would have been unthinkable to provide specific conditions, time, or space for recovery, which many ill people undoubtedly need.

The shift from rest to activity is a cultural move as much as a clinical one. In the mid nineteenth century, gravestones constantly announced eternal rest. Fatigue was a symptom that expressed social as well as clinical problems, and its remedy was rest. Hymns misquoted Jesus as offering rest to the weary, rather than refreshment.[19] Today, the dominant cultural motif is activity rather than rest. In healthcare it is not only patients who must be active; surgeons and physicians and hospitals are judged on their 'activity', which is a statistical proxy for 'product'. As Vanstone[20] says, many of us are disturbed by the idea of retirement, and by the status of invalid. We reserve our highest praise for the wonderful old person who is still cleaning the windows at 97.

The technologies of modern medicine keep both hospital staff and patients constantly busy, and the demand for medical help sends large flows of patients in and out of the wards. Psychiatric facilities have been absorbed into the same system, and there are almost no asylums, in any sense. Hospital architecture makes rest a scarce resource for most patients. A small courtyard garden may be a bolt-hole for a patient in search of peace. The hospital chapel will often have the laminated blandness of an airport's 'Faith room'. The hospital's low, plastic-panelled ceilings, clustered beds, bustling corridors, commercial outlets and air conditioning are geared for much the same kind of business as a department store. A modern hospital is a better site for the sick body than were its pre-decessors. It might be a good place for a quest narrative, but not for the meandering pathways that some people take towards wellness. Recovery, the healing process that must take its own time, is assumed to happen elsewhere. The places where community healthcare is delivered (note the commercial connotations of delivery) – for example health centres – have the same active ethos as hospitals.

The restlessly productive architecture of modern healthcare has widened the gap between disease and illness. Monastic infirmaries were suppliers of remedies and at the same time were resources for recovery, as were 19th and early 20th century hospitals and convalescent homes. The only space that still fulfils both functions today is the hospice, where death rather than life is on the horizon. Otherwise, the concept of healing has become almost an embarrassment, something that can be left to dreamers and quacks. Ill people must look elsewhere for environments where they can recover.

Interventions

When we are ill, we hope that some remedy will interrupt whatever process is causing our symptoms. Anything that has this intention is an intervention, whether it is successful or not. Whatever form they take, interventions are technologies, from the Greek word tekhnē, meaning rational practice. They are based on mechanistic knowledges, in the broad, non-pejorative sense that everything with a supposed cause also has a supposed mechanism. Based on one causal model or another, interventions always aim to effect changes in a sick person. Modern medicine offers us the technologies of surgery and pharmacology as agents of change but there are other knowledge-based efforts to eliminate or modify illness, including psychotherapy and physiotherapy and homeopathy and a vast range of other practices.

Understanding the place of interventions among other resources for recovery requires us to take a somewhat mechanistic detour here. A man I'll call Ethan was rapidly becoming paralysed because his potassium was dangerously low. Potassium depletion was due to taking a particular drug together with lots of liquorice. The causal chain was clear:

Box 9.1: Causal chain

Low potassium due to Drug + Liquorice	⇨	Lack of muscle potassium	⇨	Paralysis

Once we'd given Ethan enough potassium, he got up and walked. What could be simpler? An intervention had snipped a causal chain, just as it does when an antihistamine drug interrupts an allergic reaction or chemotherapy halts the proliferation of cancer cells. When psychotherapy targets something that is causing distress it, too, is an intervention. Homeopathy is an intervention, and so is prayer when it is a plea for a disease process to be interrupted.

The meanings of interventions often cause confusion, through a failure to recognise their rationale. A minority are designed to be curative, which is not to say that they bring about healing directly, whatever claims are made about them. Interventions to promote healing indirectly are remedial. A physiotherapist who releases a limb's reflex spasms following brain damage is supporting the natural tendency of reflex systems to rebalance themselves. A Hippocratic doctor's effort to restore the balance between the humours had a similar aim to re-establish nature's equilibrium, and so does psychotherapy. Other interventions are palliative. Although palliation derives from the Latin for cloak, palliative measures such as pain treatments soften rather than disguise illness experience.[21] A prosthetic intervention replaces something that is non-functioning. An artificial leg is a prosthetic replacement for an amputation, a memory aid for a cognitive impairment, and a transfusion blood loss.[22]

Many interventions are acts of destruction. It is difficult to see how something that modifies what was going to happen could ever be entirely safe. If we had given Ethan potassium too fast it would have killed him. Prozac has been seen by some as a cure and by others as muffling a person's reality. Psychotherapy can cause dangerous distress. It is possible for homeopathy and other alternative medical interventions to do more harm than good in situations where a different resource has a better chance of promoting healing. Interventions that lack personal meaning are usually damaging. Louise, a woman with rheumatoid arthritis, politely declined a surgeon's forceful offer to operate on her deformed hand because it was not a problem in her life. Operating on it would have been harmful. I wonder whether prayer, too, can be dangerous.

Dialogue between patients, doctors and others will promote more meaningful recovery. A shared vision of wellness is difficult to achieve. One problem is that interventions tend to proceed independently of one another, as though the patient was a customer shunting a trolley through IKEA, knowing what she is looking for. Doctors are shoppers as well. The life of a woman called Gill involved a constant struggle with a multitude of MS-related impairments, drug complications and conflicted emotions. Describing my last encounter with her in my journal[23], I saw myself as 'wandering around the interlocking problems, fingering them and then dropping them (like someone choosing a scarf on a market stall)'. I was feeling the compulsion to intervene that my nurse colleague Alison Smith calls the professional righting reflex. Worrying about making things worse, I was losing sight of Gill's own desires.

Therapeutic nihilism, the supposed virtue of doing nothing, is an opposite danger. 'Conservative' medicine can sometimes be the morally respectable face of indifference or laziness. It can also reflect a dread of taking risks on a patient's behalf. Injecting phenol into the spinal fluid makes a patient's legs flaccid and useless. It was going to be useful for Meg, a woman with severe muscle spasms due to MS, if it enabled her to sit in a wheelchair instead of being forced by her contorted posture to spend all day on a bed, but there was a possibility that it would make things disastrously worse. My blood pressure was high while I was injecting her because this was a risky act of destruction (I doubt if I could have been a surgeon).

The decision to stop treatment altogether is commonly debated by ethicists and lawyers. A much less public practice is to do less, which is often a way of doing nothing by stealth. Petra, a woman with motor neurone disease, was receiving only half-hearted treatment for her pneumonia when I visited her on a medical ward, because staff assumed that anyone with such a terrible disease would rather be dead. I protested against this since, as I knew, Petra was constantly 'recovering' a life that she valued. The problem here was that doctors and nurses were taking a standardised view of Petra rather than accessing her feelings.

Modern healthcare is often flummoxed by even small deviations from its idea of a standard patient, despite its person-centred rhetoric.

> *Bert was an elderly man with severe Parkinson's disease who happened also to have an arthrodesed (unbending) right knee following childhood TB. When Bert was hospitalised following a fall, ward staff spent the best part of a month pondering what to do about him. None of the standard therapies and procedures matched his needs. Moreover, therapists could not imagine how he could survive at home with such a strange combination of problems.*

Having visited Bert several times at home I knew he had got along quite well with the same set of difficulties for several years. Unusualness is the rule in human life, not the exception. Responding to individual needs requires imagination as well as protocols.

Matching interventions to individual desires and needs is what rehabilitation aims to do. When a derelict house is rehabilitated, we expect it to be as good as new, so it is understandable that people with long-term conditions are suspicious of the rehabilitation concept. Rehabilitation is also criticised when it seems to be urging people back to the labour market or the battlefield.[24] The word recovery is an equally misleading description of the person-centred, collaborative effort that rehabilitation aspires to, but no-one has come up with a more expressive word. Possibilitation, perhaps? In the language of contemporary healthcare, rehabilitation at least conveys the need for health services (1) to agree with their patients on the purposes of interventions and (2) to do what they can do together, rather than in isolation.

Capital

When I was a trainee physician on the admissions ward, there were patients, mostly elderly, whom we found especially perplexing and frustrating. Our private diagnosis was 'acopia', I am ashamed to say, because we thought of them as failing to cope with life's practical, mental and social demands.[25] These unfortunate people typically had little money, were socially isolated, and moreover lacked the reserve capacities that help to maintain physical, psychological and social equilibrium in times of stress. Some were more ill than others but they had one thing in common: a lack of capital. Capital in a general sense includes all the assets that a person has accumulated prior to illness, including money along with social, cultural and biological advantages.

Capital makes a vital contribution to resilience.[26] Money buys you out of certain kinds of suffering and paves the way for well-being. As is well known, wealth is linked to mortality rate across the globe.[27] Social capital, including one's network of relationships, both protects from illness and smooths the path to recovery. Cultural capital, as Bourdieu defines it, is the amalgam of habits, attitude and style – the habitus – that influences how a person is treated in healthcare settings. The reserve capacities that protect against illness or promote recovery could be called biological capital. A malnourished body heals less readily than a well-nourished one, a heart with less muscle power is more likely to fail, and someone who has suffered previous psychological trauma is less able to withstand additional stresses.

People

Human beings are irreplaceable resources for healing because they alone can care about and emphathise with an ill person.

Care

The purpose of an intervention is to change things but the aim of care is to sustain. This distinction is lost when the word care is extended to interventions ('healthcare', 'care pathways', etc). Care's most basic role is to provide for practical needs such as protection, nutrition, and hydration, thus creating the conditions for healing. During World War 2, the outlook for survivors of spinal-cord injuries was revolutionised when Dr Ludwig Guttman, founder of the Paralympics, inspired nurses, therapists and doctors to care more intensively for their patients. Medical interventions were powerless to repair the neural damage at that time, and they still are.[28]

Those injured servicemen were being better cared for but they were also being cared about. Caring-about is like love: it does not seek to change the person, as interventions do. Actions such as rearranging the pillows or refilling the water jug are forms of care similar to those of a parent soothing a distressed child. To care is to comfort the soul as well as the body. The way we want to be cared for reflects our experiences as infants.[29] A child in agonising pain cries out: 'Help me mummy!'. Even when mum cannot do much, she is valued simply for being there. Parental presence creates the pattern for all forms of care. Screams and groans would have punctuated the tranquillity of monastic infirmaries and Victorian hospitals and across today's medical and surgical wards there are still constant calls of 'Nurse! Nurse!'. Distressed patients have practical needs, but many also hope for some person to come to the bedside, if only for the comfort that human company can bring.

Trust

Research evidence shows that therapeutic outcomes are influenced by who the clinician is, as well as by what she does. It can hardly be true that surgical technique matters less than surgical charisma, but research evidence leaves little doubt that a doctor's personal characteristics influence recovery. Daniel Moerman suggests that what matters most is how the doctor communicates rather than what is said.[30] Perhaps trust is the key. Someone who is not trusted cannot reassure or console or fully empathise. My cultural capital as a physician and professor gave me a head start in encounters with patients but I still often had to work hard to be trusted. When my colleague asked Bronwen (p. 83) if she had difficulty in trusting doctors, she replied briskly: 'You're dead right I do. They got my daughter's diagnosis wrong three times'. It is difficult to win the trust of people who have felt betrayed by those who were supposed to be helping them. An atmosphere of suspicion is constantly stirred up on the internet where you will learn that 'doctors, the "priests of the Church of Modern Medicine" are in fact 'only human — in the worst ways. You can't assume your doctor is any of the nice things listed above, because doctors turn out to be dishonest, corrupt, unethical, sick, poorly educated, and downright stupid more often than the rest of society'[31].

People with contested diagnoses have 'illnesses you have to fight to get'.[32] We used to say that you'd never get better until you had persuaded people you were ill, and many of my patients wanted someone to look them in the eye and say 'I believe you'.

> *Stuart was a young man with severe head pains, subject to dramatic fits that he called 'my wobbles'. Several doctors had dismissed his symptoms as imaginary. We helped him connect his distress with a period in his childhood when he was being sexually abused by a family friend and was not believed by his father. Stuart's symptoms dramatically improved once he began to feel believed, and he also perhaps became a little less distrustful of doctors.*

The polysymptomatic patients I described in Chapter 5, who have difficulty in expressing their distress, are often 'help-deniers'[33] because they have had experiences similar to Stuart's. An experiment involving inflicting painful stimuli on healthy volunteers gives us a hint of how previous experiences of relationships might affect a person's ability to be helped by others. Some participants in the study reported less pain when an intimate partner was present. Those whose pain was not lessened by the presence of a partner were found to have a psychological profile called 'attachment avoidant', suggesting attachment problems in early life.[34] Doctors and therapists must be attuned to such differences and work to establish trust.

People sometimes make contributions to each other's recovery because shared experience creates trust. On rehabilitation units people often encourage and sometimes challenge each other. In a group of people with MS, one man's voice was dominating the conversation until another equally disabled person cheerfully chided him for his self-pity. I could never have said this, but the man accepted it from a person who had shared some of his experiences. In John Berryman's fictional account of recovery one member of an Alcoholics Anonymous group says to another 'It's true, it's true isn't it? Your life is a nightmare. You are an alcoholic pal. You are almost as sick as I am, maybe more so'.[35]

Family therapy helps people say difficult things to one another in a more regulated way.

Suffering belongs to the self and the self alone, but the mere presence of another person can be therapeutic if it reduces the intensity of this feeling. A sick child is reassured when a parent is near; Florence Nightingale, as 'the lady with the lamp', was keeping company with wounded soldiers. A book title, *Healing Presence. The Essence of Nursing* conveys one of a nurse's essential characteristics.[36] Doctors are too confident in their power to reassure. I have seen terse outpatient notes along these lines – 'Anxious about palpitations. Reassured'; 'Asked about prognosis. Reassured'; or 'I reassured her that the numbness in her hand was what we would expect . . . '. Reassurance is promoted as a technique,[37] but responding to the mistrust of a person such as Stuart requires something more.

Accompanying

A still more basic need than reassurance, felt by everyone from infancy onwards, is to be noticed. An intangible aspect of our work with long-term conditions was that we were witnesses. Even an intimate partner might miss some of the elements of illness experience that doctors and nurses see. People mostly want to hide the raw physicality of illness from the outside world, but they might nevertheless want someone to see the body's sickness as they see it themselves. This could have been the impetus behind Anatole Broyard's desire to sit down with a doctor and talk about his prostate, to 'have a meditation, a rumination, a lucubration, a bombination' about it. 'What a curious organ. What can God have been thinking when he designed it this way?'.[38]

Because I followed my patients for years on end, I accompanied them through radical changes in their bodies and lives. Adrian, whom I had known for a long time, said he thought that 'in the circumstances I am coping rather well'. Moments later a stream of urine flowed from his disconnected urine bag to the clinic floor, making me a witness to his experience of multiple sclerosis without (hopefully) being a trigger for shame. We accompanied people like Adrian in their endless engagements with chronic illness, just as a midwife accompanies a woman through labour. If we were a therapeutic resource it was because we were persons rather than technicians. This aspect of our work was unquantifiable, and invisible to our managers.

A more ambiguous form of support that people offer one another is consolation. We expect a consolation prize to compensate for something, but authentic consolation acknowledges suffering for what it is and does not claim to 'make up for it'. Consolation is a possible remedy for the irremediable. Boethius, on the Roman equivalent of death row, drew consolation from philosophy.[39] Religious writings offer the consolations of divine love, which for some people is the kind of assurance a parent or a spouse can give, that a person is valued and has meaning. The worst forms of suffering are those where a person cannot perceive any meaning in existence. Alan, the man with motor neurone disease I described in Chapter 7 (p. 78), might have been inconsolable because he could see no meaning in the life remaining to him.

Empathy

The resource on which care, understanding, witnessing, consolation and all other benefits of human help depend is empathy. A woman with motor neurone disease recalls feeling distressed when a consultant patted her on the arm, saying 'I'm sorry my dear, as I suspected, you have motor neurone disease. It's very serious, but you're an intelligent woman and I know you would like to know'.[40] The doctor imagined that touching was an empathic gesture, but he was not attuned to the woman's sensibility. We should think of empathy, like suffering, as existing only if it is experienced as such by the individual. Research suggests that outcomes of physical conditions are influenced by the degree of empathy that a doctor 'has',[41] and we speak of a doctor 'showing' empathy, but I prefer to think of empathising as a skill developed between people, like the skill of playing a duet. Skills can be increased or neglected. Medical students seem to become less empathic during their training.[42] The emotional and intellectual demands on them probably make students less open to certain kinds of relationships with their patients.

For obvious reasons, we medical students always affected indifference to the human meanings of what we saw and smelt when we first entered the dissecting room or the morgue. Three years later, wearing a white coat and a nervous smile, I was ushered on to a ward for the first time by a medical registrar who was like someone out of M★A★S★H. 'The game here is to guess which are alive and which are dead', he said. I looked down a long ward flanked by bodies beneath by starchy sheets, and wondered. The registrar pointed out 'classic cases' of common illnesses, and recommended a patient with a 'good' heart murmur. The rest of the patients, invariably the most elderly ones, were dismissed as 'crumble', a piece of demeaning medical slang that is sadly still current.[43] Honest accounts of medical life acknowledge the macabre humour that dulls empathy. Empathy is not created with a tilt of the head and a soft voice. It must flow from genuine curiosity and genuine care.

Enabling

People become agents of recovery when they sit beside someone rather than standing in front, blocking the light. A nurse who is truly interested in a person's suffering enables it to be expressed, unlike one who shunts her drug trolley into a four-bedded ward and shouts 'Any pain anyone?' (This happened when I was a patient myself, recovering from a minor operation. The man in the next bed was riddled with cancer, so I kept quiet about my own pain, even though I was miserable). I have watched a husband waiting for his wife to find her own words rather than speaking for her, just as a physiotherapist will enable someone to walk safely, not touching the body, but ready to prevent a fall.

> *Dick, a man with Huntington's disease, is an unlikely illustration of how other people can enable a person to flourish in a protective environment. Every morning at about 4.30 am he wobbled precariously towards the newsagent on his bike, obsessively determined to be the first with the day's news. As often as not a police car would sidle up and follow him at a distance, making sure he did not tip into the traffic. Dick was probably unaware that he was being cared for (and cared about) by anyone, let alone a cop.*

The idea of enabling environments, which is familiar in education, resonates with modern concepts of disability and extends seamlessly into the domain of illness. Vygotsky conceived of the 'zone of proximal development' as a protected space within which a child could explore the world as freely as possible. A person requires a similar environment for recovery.[44] No external resource is enough, however. Change can only happen if the alcoholic takes a first step, or the man with a stroke makes a first attempt to communicate, or the dying person does or says or feels something. The next chapter is about the personal resources that make it possible to be less ill.

Notes

1 Stacey 1988, Chapter 1
2 Warrell et al. 2010
3 See Cutter 2011, preface by M Prince: in the ancient rabbinical Samuel midrash there is a story of a vineyard worker claiming that offering medical help is meddling in God's business. The sages (rabbis) ask why he meddles in God's work in his vineyard. 'If I didn't go out and plough the vineyard, prune it, compost it, and weed it, it would yield nothing'. 'The human body is a tree' say the sages, 'a healing potion is the compost, and the physician is the tiller of the soil'
4 Mental health charities view recovery as distinct from psychiatric interventions (see Mind https://bit.ly/2JkSxIp and Rethink https://bit.ly/2XevvIp)

5 The Bible. Luke 18:42
6 These etymological points might reflect the biases of philologists (it being hard to know how ancient words worked in their own contexts), but if so, they reflect a nexus of ideas about wholeness and saving that is relevant at least in European cultures
7 Zautra et al. 2010. I will say more about resilience in Chapter 10.
8 Wong et al. 2013
9 See Curth 2003
10 Hilton 1863/1950
11 Coryllos PN, 1933
12 Mitchell 1899, Chapter 5
13 Mann 1928
14 See a series of papers in *Journal of the History of Medicine and Allied Sciences*, 73:127–205, 2018
15 Martin 2016
16 See Noga Arikha's excellent history of the humours (2007)
17 Ulrich 1984.
18 See Anders 2014, and for a premodern version of convalescence Newton 2017
19 See Ward 2008
20 Vanstone 1982
21 From the Latin for soft, how about 'molliative care'?
22 To complete this typology of interventions, orthoses straighten out deformities
23 Clinical incidents described in my private journal are thoroughly anonymised
24 Leplège et al. 2015
25 Oliver 2008
26 Smith & Hayslip 2012
27 For example, Holder, 2018: BBC analysis shows that the rate of avoidable deaths is three to four times higher in the poorest and wealthiest parts of the UK; Australian Institute of Health and Welfare, 2018. www.bbc.co.uk/news/uk-england-44853482
28 See Sir Ludwig Guttman. Obituary by AK Thomas, *BMJ*, April 5 1980. www.bmj.com/content/280/6219/1021
29 Conversely the urge to care – for good or ill – has a connection with whatever makes parents of us
30 For reviews of the influence of clinicians on outcomes see Horvarth & Luborsky 1993 and Lambert & Barley 2001 on psychotherapy; Kelley et al. 2014 on other healthcare; and Moerman 20012, Chapter 4, on the doctor's personality and communicative style; Thomas 1987 is an example of a GP-based study.
31 Church of Allopathy *The Devil's Priests* By Robert S. Mendelsohn, M.D. Chapter 7: [1991] Confessions of a Medical Heretic Doc (www.whale.to/c/devilspriests.html)
32 'Illnesses you have to fight to get' – Dumit 2006
33 The phrase comes from Groves 1978, a very medical perspective on difficult patients.
34 Krahé et al. 2015; for suggested links between borderline personality disorder and attachment difficulties see Fonagy 2000
35 Berryman 1973, IV – The Last Two Steps
36 Koerner 2011. Unfortunately, the author provides few person-based examples of what presence is, either for the nurse or the patient
37 Kathol 1997
38 Broyard 1992, p. 52
39 Boethius. *The Consolation of Philosophy*. c. 524
40 Allen-Collinson & Pavey 2014
41 Mercer et al. 2016; Derksen et al 2013
42 Hojat et al. 2009
43 Known as 'crumblies' according to Oliver 2008
44 Holaday et al. 1994

10

ABILITIES

Chapter 9 surveyed resources that the world offers to an ill person. This one is about the strengths and abilities that help a person survive illness. Triumph over adversity is one of the great Hollywood themes but most of us have encountered real people who overcome stresses in extraordinary ways. I think of 18-year-old Françoise, a few weeks after a car accident while on holiday in this country, curled up in a hospital bed. She had emerged from a long coma but was still strangely stiff and unresponsive. She puzzled us neurologically, and from a rehabilitation point of view we could not feel hopeful. She was in a neurological state called abulia, in which desires and initiative vanish. But I also have another image of her, a photo taken after returning home many months later. She is seated in a wheelchair, wearing a bright green anorak. She is earning a living, and flourishing. Then there is Matteo – whose motor neurone disease had made him nearly helpless (what an odd word: 'helpless'). Matteo's flaccid laryngeal muscles would have made his speech difficult for me to understand even without his strong Italian accent, but you knew you were in the presence of a spirit that refused to be snuffed out by illness. Matteo also refused not to laugh at life. He always maintained that what he found hardest was worrying about his wayward daughter Sophia. Compared to this, he insisted, motor neurone disease was 'a walk on the beach', although it had been months since he had walked even across a room. I also think of Lucy. Years ago, she attacked her wrist in a savage effort to kill herself. She has carried physical scars ever since and also, I am sure, psychological ones, but she has found her way out of the pit of depression and has lived a life that has been creative, generous and sometimes happy.

The concept of resilience spread from its origins in studies of neglected and abused children to include elderly adults and survivors of human disasters. It easily leads to the idea that what a person brings to the problem of illness is a set of positive character traits, but I will argue that recovery, or being less ill, depends more on skills than on fixed attributes.

Resilience

When it comes to displaying resilience, most people are like the children of Lake Wobegon, all of whom are above average. Ann Masten's lovely phrase 'ordinary magic' refers to the well evidenced observation that most children who have adverse experiences eventually continue their development more or less success-fully,[1] just as the majority of adults are able to resume their lives in the wake of war, natural disasters and other traumas. I have witnessed ordinary magic in an extraordinary number of people. Husbands or wives, as carers of their spouses, often quoted their marriage vows to me: '. . . for better for worse, for richer for poorer, in sickness and in health . . .'.[2] Diane, who used to say 'spit on your hands and get on with it', came from a former mining community and her words sug-gested the image of shovelling coal, which would be a good metaphor for the way many people endure progressive illness. No sooner had one crisis hit Diane than another shovelful of difficulties came her way, but she never seemed to give up. Survival was the only option. Diane was typical of many people whom I saw in terrible situations. When I asked her how she managed to 'carry on', she said 'You have to, don't you?'. Freud, being told that a severely disabled man was admirably heroic, asked 'What else can he do?'.[3]

We hardly need research evidence, although there is plenty of it, to know that well-being is critically dependent on 'attitude'.[4] Anyone's list of positive attitudes would include insight, wisdom, self-control and self-confidence. Ivan Illich imagi-nes 'traditional peoples' keeping themselves well with 'patience, forbearance, courage, resignation, self-control, perseverance and meekness',[5] recalling the Apostle Paul's 'patience, kindness, goodness, faithfulness, gentleness, self-control'.[6] Aristotle recommended many of these as the essential virtues of eudaimonia. Par-ticularly valuable, in illness, is the positivity that enables you to see the funny side in the worst of situations, and to see a crisis as an opportunity to grow.[7]

If people rise to the challenges of illness in wonderful ways, as funeral eulogies and obituaries would have us believe, why are there those who do not 'bounce back'? Must we think of them as lacking capacities that 'normal' individuals have? Research on resilience and on happiness sometimes suggests that we should. Many of the items I listed earlier as the ingredients of resilience are items in personality questionnaires, implying that they are more or less fixed traits. There is evidence that at least some aspects of them are partly heritable.[8] Viewed as a trait, 'bounce' would appear to be one that most people have.

The trait perspective on resilience has a corollary, that if illness knocks you flat it is because you are an inadequate person. Normal people ought always to be able produce ordinary magic, it seems. John Diamond, in the midst of his own cancer, comments drily that a five-year-old with leukaemia is always 'brave little Linda'.[9] People who appear to be making heavy weather of illness are sometimes thought to be defective, because they lack insight, humour or confidence. Little Linda might perhaps be classed as inadequate, or even given a diagnosis of some sort, if her bravery did not meet expectations. Cognitive styles such as catastrophising, over-thinking and pessimism, and the tendency to locate the causes of difficulties in the outside world rather than in oneself (so-called external attributions) can be framed as failures, as though independence of thought and action were the norm. Behind closed doors, doctors will describe a 'difficult' patient in terms of character defects. As medical trainees we would borrow the cheerful but chilling military humour of the time, dubbing someone 'N.O.M' – not officer material; or 'L.M.F' – low moral fibre.

There is something wrong with a concept of resilience that attributes people's chances of recovery to whether they are either wonderful or awful characters. The problem comes into focus in a recent scientific think-piece that recommends ageing mice as an animal model with which to 'test resilience accurately and predictably'.[10] The vision here is of resilience as something inside you, a resource that would be good to 'have' when you are under threat. Gregory Bateson, a pioneer of human systems ideas, would call resilience a dormitive concept[11] when it produces this syllogism:

People (and also mice) who have good outcomes are resilient
People (and mice) who are resilient have resilience
Resilience gives you (or a mouse) a good outcome

Think of a suspension bridge, which as said in the last chapter will 'bounce back' when a gust of wind hits it; and think of a human being, recovering gradually or rapidly from some external stress. It would be true to say that each of these is a system with resilience – with 'bounce' – but 'bounce' is not a thing that either the bridge or the person contains. It describes a set of relationships within the system's elements (between, say, the suspension cables and the bridge's supporting framework; or between the cognitive and emotional responses that a traumatic experience produces in a person). Bounce also, of course, defines the relationship of the system as a whole with the wind, in the case of a bridge, or with external stressors in the case of a person.

Survival skills

The defect perspective is discouraging to those who are overwhelmed by illness, and it breeds therapeutic pessimism among their helpers. A more hopeful possibility is that resilience depends on skills.[12] Skill is a quality, not a thing. Human performances as diverse as throwing and thinking are skilful to the extent that the elements in the body's system are in ideal relationships with one another, as when the tilt of a footballer's boot is just right, or a comedian times the punchline perfectly. A person's innate traits do contribute to skilled performance (it is better to have long fingers if you are a pianist) but practice is essential. 'Emotional regulation', in psychological jargon, is a skill that is acquired over time – no-one is born with it - and that often fails in times of stress. Cognitive behavioural therapy is one way of increasing this skill, and mindfulness training is another. Imagination, humour and glass-half-full positivity depend on the skill of seeing things in new ways. No new-born infant has those abilities. Categorising people as 'dependent clingers', 'entitled demanders', 'manipulative help-rejecters' and 'self-destructive deniers'[13] is a negative way of saying that their efforts to get help are unskilful.

Denial

One of the skills for wellness is the ability to manage one's 'spoiled identity'.[14] A speckless house and smart clothes protect you from being thought anything less than heroic. Since unregulated feelings make enemies, the skill of controlling one's emotional outbursts is worth having from a purely social point of view, just as it is easier to make friends and get support if one has the skill of appearing to be positive and appearing to be grateful. Social skills protect us from being labelled as difficult patients. Since they are a means for illness to be performed effectively (Chapter 5) and to be understood by others (Chapter 6), they are also resources for recovery. They are useful 'technologies of the self', to use Foucault's language.[15]

It is good to put a brave face on things, people think, but a bad thing to deny reality. And yet, denial is a useful skill. Toddlers are slow to learn that politeness involves skilful denials: think how we teach our children not to stare. As AL Kennedy said[16], death is something you generally have to look at out of the corner of your eye, which makes denying it trickier, but Ernest Becker is right that we do deny it, almost constantly.[17] In times of crisis, denial can be a source of strength rather than a sign of weakness. 'Spitting on your hands and getting on with it' may only be possible if certain realities are evaded, at least for the time being.

> *Sinaid and Jock (as I'll call them) told me that when the doctor first told them that Sinaid's leg weakness was due to MS, they came out of the consulting room in silence and said not another word about the fateful diagnosis for a full three months.*

We need not think of Sinaid and Jock's denial as a defect. They were mustering the skills to carry on with their lives in the face of an almost unbearable threat. If Becker's death-denying story is correct, we are all doing the same thing, all the time.

Almost everyone knows that death is a matter of fact, but we often behave as though it was not, so that it would be more correct to say that we disavow rather than deny it. Jock and Sinaid may have been disavowing MS. Disavowal can be a more or less unconscious process.[18] Elaine's blindness and Wahid's leg paralysis (pp. 48–49), probably both stood for some distress that had been hidden more completely. Their 'unspeakable dilemmas' had been made bearable by being 'walled off' from consciousness. This is the process that Freud called repression, and that has affinities with Pierre Janet's concept of dissociation.[19] The walling off of traumatic experiences is useful because it enables a person to function from day to day, even if it causes negative consequences at some point in the future. Denial and its unconscious variants are not signs of a defective personality or a weak character. On the contrary, they are part of everyday life, as Freud showed.[20] The ability to dissociate from aspects of reality probably depends in some degree on hardwired physiological mechanisms,[21] but it is also an unconsciously practised skill that contributes to some people's resilience more than to others'.

Becker calls 'death transcendence' a knack or a skill that explains our 'normal cultural heroism' and our 'easy yielding to the superordinate cultural world-view'. Normal cultural heroism is a description of the world of symbols and ideas and aspirations that we build despite our utterly unheroic bodies. It is a form of ordinary magic. Becker goes so far as to claim that mental illness is the failure of that ability.[22]

Acceptance

A more conventional skill to consider is acceptance. My aunt Doris, a model of resilience, died at the age of 105. 'Acceptance is peace' was her mantra. True acceptance is incompatible with denial. It requires an unflinching affirmation of reality, however unpleasant. According to Melanie Klein, the developing infant must abandon the 'schizoid-paranoid' position in which unbridled fantasy is possible, in favour of what she depressingly calls the depressive position, which is able to deal with the possibility that one's self and one's parents and one's world have limitations.[23]

A word my patients sometimes used was stoicism. The meaning of stoicism can be debased to the cheery 'mustn't grumble' positivity that comedian Alexei Sayle used to parody, or the somewhat irritating 'smiling and whistling under all difficulties' that Baden-Powell recommended. However, stoicism can also stand for the radiant resilience of a Sinaid or a Matteo. Stoics accept that some things are beyond their control. Reinhold Niebuhr's celebrated prayer, familiar to the 12-Step Programme of Alcoholics Anonymous, is a call for wisdom in distinguishing between what can and cannot be changed.[24] Wisdom is an acquired skill, as any person, and any parent, knows. It is not a fixed faculty.

Acceptance is a tight-rope between apathy and creative resistance. Apathy is not the only risk: another danger is to struggle pointlessly with unchangeable reality. Someone with chronic illness will probably be held back from acceptance by a picture of health as perfection, and helped towards it by an ability to think of health as 'tolerant of ill health'; or even to follow Winnicott still further, imagining that 'health gains much from being in touch with ill health with all its aspects', which is a far cry from the WHO's definition.[25] Repunctuating disease as a normal phenomenon (see p. 24) produces the Stoic idea that even the worst of things are natural. Aristotle would describe walking the tight-rope of acceptance as a virtue – a skilled practice - that contributes to a good life. Ill-being intensifies the need for such skills.

Acceptance of the tight-rope variety is not passive; it is not resignation - it is compatible with hope. Life is meaningless without hopes and desires, but there are unhappy hopers, and desire can be torment. Everything hinges on active rather than passive expectation. To expect is to look out for something.[26] Someone who complacently expects either a cure or its opposite is likely to be an unhappy hoper. A person who actively accepts what she is experiencing can at the same time hopefully expect – look for – a better form of life. One's desires and hopes must not be abandoned but they do need winnowing. Some are toxic, as Buddhists know. Restitution narratives and quest narratives can often be driven by an 'aggressive, object-seeking desire', but this type of desire 'awakens the mind to the impossibility of its demands . . . [and]. pushes it to explore the uncharted territory of its own dissatisfactions'.[27] In another direction I know there are satisfactions to be found even among people whom the world regards as 'hopeless cases' from a medical point of view, because I saw people find them.

This is the place to say something more about illnesses you have to fight to get (see p. 108). You can only follow the orthodox path towards recovery if you have secured a foothold, which people with contested diagnoses can never achieve if the struggle to persuade others that they are ill produces a form of acceptance that entrenches them in illness. Getting better will involve a shift in how they view their symptoms, an ability to 'perform' their distress in ways that others can understand (as described in Chapter 5), and a measure of resistance to the habitus of illness that culture prescribes.

Disobedience

One way of escaping illness is to disobey the rules of illness and wellness. Throwing off the habitus of illness and finding a different way of conceptualising your wellness might require the skill of reimagining both your predicament and your desires. I think Pierre Bourdieu would be pessimistic about your chances of doing this because he sees human agency as entirely bound up with social practices.[28] Have I seen anyone do it? Hypnosis gave Wahid (p. 49) a dignified exit from illness that did not require any skill on his part (on the contrary, his narrative of cure might have encouraged his reliance on similar interventions to solve any future troubles).

People certainly rebel in an opposite way, not against illness but against an accepted image of betterness. Cheryl (pp. 93–94) preferred to be looked after rather than following the prescribed route towards independence. It takes skill as well as courage to make a stand (or rather to stay sitting) as Cheryl did. I have given plenty of examples of people in whom the ability to be well on their own terms was the corollary of their individual images of 'ill-ness'. Matteo was 'doing' motor neurone disease in his own way, as a walk on the beach. Gwyneth and her husband Mick (pp. 101–102) chose walking, at any cost, rather than the smoother form of wellness offered by a wheelchair existence. In a way, they were staying with illness of a kind in order to have wellness. Stuart (p. 108) regained enough trust in other people to see his symptoms in the light of a traumatic past history. Psychotherapy supported Stuart's skill in letting go of an image of himself as physically sick and disabled, to the extent that he was able to find a job for the first time in years. In my experience the skill of denial is often involved in this kind of recovery. I am thinking of two young women with functional weakness, each of whom was entrenched in a view of herself as a wheelchair-dependent invalid. In their different ways they gradually moved, literally out of their wheelchairs and metaphorically from illness towards less constraining existences. Neither of them wanted to talk about exactly what the original problem was, or about exactly how she recovered. There is a certain skilful grace in the way people leave such questions aside in order to get on with their lives.

Meaning

The survival skills I have described – denial, acceptance and disobedience – are held together by an ability to stay in touch with personal meanings. Denial and acceptance can each have a numbing effect unless they clear a path towards something that an ill person positively desires. A lively sense of what matters – a vision of wellness - is the necessary spur to disobedience. Viktor Frankl describes the vital importance of finding a point in life even in the direst circumstances.[29] I will say more about this shortly.

Reflection

Illnesses and injury always play havoc with assumptions. It might simply be that you have to ditch your plans for the day because you are vomiting; or that putting your foot to the ground is suddenly a problem, as Oliver Sacks found; or that things you thought you knew well escape you, as they did Wendy Mitchell in her dementia.[30] If you lose your bearings, as you may do in illness, perhaps you begin to talk to yourself, as when Pessoa wonders whether a chasm in the self is physical, or mental, or neither (p. 94). A traumatic moment is often the trigger for an inner conversation. Audre Lorde writes that following her encounter with breast cancer there was a background of 'pain and terror and disbelief' in which she could hear 'a thin high voice . . . screaming that none of this was true, it was all a bad dream that would go away if I became totally inert'. Tom Lubbock documents his reflections in a similar situation. 'I've always found . . . that my self restores itself', he writes. 'I had in me this comic spirit of immortality. Now I feel nothing, though perhaps this will return'. The crisis often provokes an effort after meaning. When Anatole Broyard was told he had cancer, 'it was like an immense electric shock. I felt galvanized. I was a new person. All my old trivial selves fell away, and I was reduced to essence'. Porochista Khakpour, musing on her symptoms, wonders 'if something else was going on. Was it the pill? My injured brain? Was something off on a deeper level?'. We make vows to ourselves at such times, for example Audre Lorde's intention, following her diagnosis to 'tend my body with at least as much care as I tend the compost . . . '. John Diamond ponders how to square the 'jauntiness' of his *Times* column with whatever his own cancer might mean. 'Normally I try to address any qualms I have about what I'm about to write before I sit down and write it. This time, I'm sorry, I can't. There you are: the truth at last'. More general meanings come into view at the same time. Speaking to herself, in her journal, Katherine Mansfield contemplates tuberculosis: 'Now Katherine, what do you mean by health? And what do you want it for?'[31] Published narratives provide dramatisations, akin to Shakespearian soliloquies, of dialogues with the self. Even when we are truly alone, we may, as Proust says, speak 'without meaning what we say, as we talk to a stranger'[32]; we might be just 'making conversation', playing with possible ways of seeing and saying things, but the skill of doing this is nevertheless a part of recovery.

A person's inner monologue is rarely disclosed to a doctor. In an email to a friend, Ruth Picardie says she does not want to talk about her cancer with 'the sad, bald fucks you meet in hospital all the time'.[33] I did sometimes hear snatches of someone's ruminations, however. A young man with progressively disabling MS told me he wondered if he had accepted his plight too much. Should he have fought more? The question was addressed more to himself than to me, I thought. When Adrian reported that 'I think I've done rather well in the circumstances', he was probably examining himself. Sinaid gave few hints of what was going on in her head in the weeks after her diagnosis but the way she and Jock withstood the repeated onslaughts of MS during the years I knew them convinced me that things had, as it were, been 'said' in conversations with herself.

Illness tests assumptions that go to the core of a person's being: for Islam, illness is not a punishment from Allah but a test.[34] 'Before, after' writes Tom Lubbock of his diagnosis. 'The present wipes out the preceding. What before was possible, and kept from clear sight, is now absolute, irrevocable. And the other possibilities are out of sight . . . '.[35] I had the brutal experience, as a neurology trainee, of explaining that weakness and wasting in a man's thumb muscles was due to motor neurone disease. He raised his hands and contemplated them silently before softly protesting, I think more to himself than to me: 'I'm a carpenter. That's my living'. He would have gone on talking to himself, I imagine, for weeks or months or years following this moment.

Illness reminds you of the strange fact that you are not alone, as Proust puts it[36] – you have a body. The body usually hovers in the distance like a well-trained waiter, but it butts in when illness strikes, standing too close and refusing to be ignored or denied. Awareness of body can be a harrowing experience in even the most trivial of illnesses, but awareness of death is worse. Illness topples your death-denying heroism and suggests, however faintly, that you are mortal. Cancer implies to Audre Lorde that 'I am not supposed to exist. I carry death around in my body like a condemnation. But I do live. The bee flies. There must be some way to integrate death into living, neither ignoring it nor giving in to it'.[37]

The very largest of moral and metaphysical issues become personal in illness, which injects urgency into questions that previously seemed remote and academic. What you mean by your self, as distinct from your body, becomes a difficulty that threatens to undermine your sense of integrity. Siri Hustvedt, meditating on her symptoms, asks 'Who are we, anyway? What do I actually know about myself? . . . What is body and what is mind? Is each of us a singular being or a plural one?'[38]. I have noticed that sufferers from medically questionable symptoms sometimes feel impelled to reflect on the relationship between mind and body.

In case this kind of talk sounds overblown, listen to Anatole Broyard's heartfelt desire – as absurd as it is touching – 'to discuss my prostate with my urologist not as a diseased organ but as a philosopher's stone'. He wants the meanings of his bodily experience to reach far beyond illness itself. Recovering from cancer, Rebecca Loncraine finds herself in 'open conversation' with the sky.[39] A feeling of mortality can be frightening. A sense of creatureliness connects us with problems we can safely leave to philosophers and theologians when we are well.[40] Loncraine reports that she is 'beginning to feel more grounded in natural processes. It is a relief, because a painful sense of being unnatural grew in me after my cancer diagnosis'.[41] Ruth Picardie emails a friend with a request to read more Primo Levi or Anne Frank: 'Am particularly interested in how holocaust victims contemplated death (she said melodramatically)'.[42] I have known that melodrama in much less critical situations, because there is a disturbing seriousness in even minor forms of suffering.

People who grapple with the large questions that illness raises are practical philosophers. The attitudes they adopt are not built-in traits. They are achievements, built through experiences of life, and especially of adversity, that correspond closely to the precepts of ancient philosophers. Ordinary people with motor neurone disease, for example, or MS, often develop the approach that Epictetus, the 1st–2nd century CE stoic, is recommending here:

A: 'Tell your secrets'
B: 'I say not a word, for this is under my control'
A: 'But I will fetter you'
B: 'What is that you say man? Fetter me? My leg you will fetter, but my moral purpose not even Zeus has power to overcome'
A: 'I will throw you into prison'
B: 'My paltry body rather!'
A: 'I will behead you'
B: 'Well, when did I ever tell you that mine was the only neck that could not be severed?'[43]

Sinaid might have said 'MS can have my legs, but it can't have me!'. Matteo was saying that motor neurone disease could not have his voice. The key point, according to Epictetus, is that one can change some things but not others. My patients would often say this with a sigh, as though it was a mantra that needed to be rehearsed. These are lessons, says Epictetus, that philosophers ought indeed 'to rehearse . . . write down daily' and they ought to 'exercise themselves', just as one must exercise a skill. I suspect that Sinaid was exercising in just this way, as was Diane in her shovelling, and couples' repeated affirmations of 'for better and for worse' probably reflected a pattern of continuing practice rather than a once-and-for-all decision.

According to both Pierre Hadot and Michel Foucault[44], practices of the kind Epictetus recommended were integral to ancient western philosophy. By calling them spiritual exercises, Hadot draws attention to the role of imagination and sensibility along with ideas. The people I have been quoting here were exercising their imaginations and sensibilities skilfully. Today, an ill person will often study the internet, ponder advice that has been offered, re-examine life and look for ways of 'pulling oneself together'. An ancient prescription for spiritual exercises follows the same pattern under six Greek headings: zetesis (enquiry, questioning, debate), skepsis (examination, observation, consideration, investigation), anagnosis (reading, knowledge), akroasis (listening), prosoche (attention) and enkrateia (self-mastery).[45]

The practical philosophy of illness takes many cultural forms. The skill of mindfulness, much prized by both religious and non-religious people today, involves a struggle with the self, if 'self' is how one chooses to name the locus of what one needs or wants as a person, and of what is threatened in illness. An ancient Sanskrit text on Ayurvedic medicine, the Charaka Saṃhitaā, recommends that in illness one should seek knowledge of self (aātman) in relation to knowledge of location (deṣa), knowledge of family (kula), knowledge of time (kaāla), knowledge of strength (bala), and knowledge of ability (ṣakti).[46] A Buddhist might conceptualise the self in a different way, but, as I argued in Chapter 4 (pp. 37–38), the challenge of illness will still involve taking a position regarding the self and illness. In Islam, illness is interpreted in terms of the self's relationship with Allah; balance is an important aspect of wellness.[47] In the Jewish tradition, an individual's trouble is always situated within the experience of a community, in fact of a nation, in a scheme that links 'God, Torah [biblical and other Jewish scripture] and Israel', so that traditional interpretative practices of midrash are brought to bear on illness experience with a much wider context in view.[48] The forms that reflections on illness take are clearly diverse, and my understanding of cultural variation is superficial. However, I think it is safe to assume that suffering individuals use reflection as a skilled practice in their efforts to find a way towards whatever visions of wellness they have.

Insight

New insights can take a long time to evolve but they sometimes seem to appear in a flash.

I expected a young man I'll call Joe to be embroiled in his nonspecific pains and disabling lassitude forever, and I was wondering what I hoped to achieve by meeting him in my clinic. When he reappeared one morning, however, he was a transformed man. I had been privately depressed at the thought of meeting him again, and I asked him what he imagined I was thinking when I saw his name on my list. Joe said: 'I think you would have groaned. You would have said "Oh no, not him again"'. This bold guess made us both smile. Joe told me that he had been reflecting on his life and had had a glimpse of how things could be better.

This was a volte-face, a turning away from illness. Another abrupt transformation was Hugh:

Hugh's crippling chronic pain had exhausted most medical and surgical options. Even the tiniest activities were impossible, he insisted. He came to the next appointment with startling news. He had washed the car. At a particular moment, without any apparent prior thinking, he stood up, went outside and did the job. Never has a carwash given more satisfaction.

For both these men, some new perspective had transformed the inconceivable into the achievable. A change in position, for example from passive illness to active wellness, can reveal a new view of a situation, and the reverse is also true. In systemic terms, positioning is a dynamic process.[49] I doubt if either Joe or Hugh had consciously studied their situation in the Stoic manner but what they achieved was nevertheless the liberating vision that philosophers and mystics strive for.

Many of the realities of disease are 'things I cannot change'. You can't be talked out of agonising pain, and a 'positive mental attitude' will not restore your hearing or your cognitive powers or your physical abilities, but the ability to live in any situation will be influenced by the possibilities that you can perceive. Among the three people with motor neurone disease that I described in Chapter 7, Yvonne could see a way of living 'successfully' with motor neurone disease, but Alan and Eva could not. Denis (p. 76), could not accept any form of wellness unless he was physically independent. He seems to have seen his MS in a very different way from Meg, the woman whose injection I mentioned in the last chapter (p. 106). After many active years following her injection, she nearly died from overwhelming infection. She described recovering consciousness as the infection receded. 'I thought I was dead, but I realised I was still alive when my legs didn't move'. Her ability to laugh about this, and to make us laugh, was a powerful reminder that recovery can transcend physical limitations.

Wellness for Alan, Eva and Denis might have been possible had they not been dominated by narratives that prescribed what motor neurone disease or MS were supposed to be like and how a person was supposed to cope with them. But perhaps narrative is not the right word. Illness creates pictures. In chronic illness you might see nothing but an abyss or a fog. Perhaps the idea of MS makes you see someone in a wheelchair rattling a collecting tin. When cancer is mentioned maybe you see 'fronded capillaries swamped by tumours'[50], or a prospect of endless hospital visits and intravenous drips opening up; or maybe your body anticipates pain, and shudders. Such imagery occupies the centre of your attention. You never see something in two ways at the same time: a frightening picture extinguishes a hopeful one just as surely as disgust destroys desire.[51] It takes imagination and courage – and perhaps a little help – to replace one image with another. I hope that this book's 'experiments in thinking about medicine'[52] will enable someone to see illness and wellness in new ways.

Hope

Hope is a good note on which to end. Unhappy hoping, as I described it earlier, is a sort of covert despair that inhibits recovery. On the other hand there is hope which, as the family therapist Kaethe Weingarten describes it, is less concerned with pragmatic outcomes than with an 'expression of who one wants to be and how one wants to act in the world'. This reasonable kind of hope 'does not struggle against an uncertain, unknowable future, but rather embraces it as its best bet'.[53] The same could be said of the orientation that Viktor Frankl describes in *Man's Search for Meaning*, towards thinking of one's life, in even the worst of circumstances, as having a point.[54] Meaning kindles hope, and hope keeps alive the sense of purpose that makes life worth living. In Christian theology hope is a virtue, or a practice, rather than an inborn personality trait of the kind that optimism and humour are often imagined to be.

Reasonable hope adjusts itself to what seems possible, which from a therapeutic point of view is invaluable, as Weingarten shows. A review of twenty qualitative studies on older people with chronic illnesses confirms that, at times, hope involves scaling down expectation.[55] I have often seen people fixing their hopes on small and ordinary things. But ordinary things are far from trivial, according to both Frankl and Weingarten: they are the stuff of recovery just as they are the texture of suffering. The hopes of people like Diane, and Pat and her husband Don (p. 85) could be thought of as banal, and yet heroic. However, life can sometimes be made more possible by hope that seems, for practical purposes, unreasonable. This was the kind of hope that, in Emily Dickinson's words, perched in the soul; it was to be heard in 'the chillest land – And on the strangest Sea – Yet – never – in Extremity, – It asked a crumb – of me'.[56]

Time is an important issue for Weingarten's conception of hope, and for Frankl's. Hope must in some sense transcend present sufferings. The hoping that emerges from the research quoted above is future-oriented, as are most Jewish, Christian and Islamic versions of hope. These traditions are also able to imagine hope outside time, however, as is Buddhism.[57] An ability to have hope in the moment, for that moment, is surely the secret of resilience.

Notes

1 Masten 2001
2 From the Anglican marriage vows: 'To have and to hold from this day forward, for better for worse, for richer for poorer, in sickness and in health, to love and to cherish, till death us do part'. Book of Common Prayer 1662
3 Becker 1973, p. 102

4 See for example Aldwin & Igarashi 2012

5 Illich 1976, p. 134

6 The Bible. Galatians 5: 22–23, English Standard Version

7 Psychological research on resilience and well-being produces few surprises. It would be odd if a sense of humour, or an ability to see your life as meaningful, did *not* help you in times of trouble.

8 Power & Pluess 2015

9 Diamond, p. 71

10 Kirkland et al. 2016

11 Bateson 2002, p. 80.

12 I am influenced by Ben Furman's attention to the therapeutic meaning of skills. (Furman 2010)

13 Groves 1978

14 See Goffman 1968; Griffith & Ryan 2015

15 Foucault 1988

16 Interview *Observer* Nov 11, 2018

17 Becker 1973

18 A good account of disavowal is Weintrobe 2013, Chapters 1 and 3, on attitudes to climate change

19 One can picture repressed feelings being stuffed into a compost heap where they may be 'converted' into symptoms. Dissociated feelings are simply walled off. Displacing unwelcome feelings produces what are called secondary gains.

20 Freud 2002

21 Krause-Utz & Elzinga 2018

22 Becker 1973, p. 102

23 Klein 1952

24 Attributed to the theologian Reinhold Niebuhr: 'God give me the serenity to accept the things I cannot change, courage to change the things I can, and wisdom to know the difference'

25 Winnicott 1990, p. 81

26 Latin ex, out + spectare, look. 'Et expecto resurrectionem mortuorum' in the Christian Nicene creed – 'We look for the resurrection of the dead' in the Anglican and American Episcopal translations

27 Epstein 2006, p. 182

28 For Bourdieu, the logic of practical life comprises 'actions that are reasonable without being the product of a reasoned design . . . intelligible and coherent without springing from an intention of coherence and a deliberate decision' (1990, p. 50–51)

29 Frankl 1964

30 Sacks 1986; Mitchell 2017

31 Lorde 1980, Introduction and Chapter 2; Lubbock 2012, p. 128; Broyard 1992, p. 37–38; Khakpour 2018, Chapter 4; Diamond 1998, p. 50–51; Mansfield 2006, p. 250

32 Proust 1920/1982, Part I Chapter 1

33 Picardie 1988, p. 6. I wince, being a male doctor with thin hair.

34 Ahmed 2000

35 Lubbock 2012, p. 37

36 Proust 1920/1982, Part I Chapter 1

37 Lorde 1980, Introduction

38 Hustvedt 2011, p. 69

39 Broyard 1992, p. 54; Loncraine 2018, quoting Sylvia Plath

40 'Creatureliness' is Becker's word (1973, p. 87)

41 Loncraine 2018, Chapter 4

42 Picardie 1998, p. 86–87.

43 Epictetus 2nd century CE/1956, Vol 1, p. 13

44 Foucault 1988; Hadot 1995

45 Hadot 1995, p. 81, 84. The list is from Philo Judeaus 'Who is the heir of divine things'

46 Cerulli & Brahmadathan 2009
47 Ahmed 2000; Ashy 1999
48 Weiss 2011
49 Harré 2009; see Chapter 8
50 Lewis 2010
51 Some find it impossible to 'see' a sexual partner with a urinary catheter as attractive.
52 'The Patient Examines the Doctor' in Broyard 1992
53 Weingarten 2010
54 Frankl 1964
55 Duggleby et al. 2012
56 Emily Dickinson 'Hope is the Thing with Feathers', 1861
57 Dunlap 2016

11

A DOCTOR'S NOTE

With illness experience rather than the facts of disease at its centre, this book has raised a question for me, and possibly for you. What is a doctor for, beyond the management of disease? I have been making a distinction between Scene 1, where unwellness is first felt, and Scene 2, in which a person 'offers' the idea of illness to someone like me (or you).[1] The medical encounter is a version of Scene 2. Kirmayer[2] envisions an encounter in which the doctor's overall aim is 'to subdue or settle the issue, seeking coherence'. The patient's aim is 'to break through, seeking relief'. In what circumstances, Kirmayer asks, 'does one person's coherence become another person's relief?' There are times when 'settling' someone's difficulties can take a simple, problem-solving approach. In some situations, however, especially in chronic or incurable illness, the settling process must go further than technical explanations and interventions.

An influential model of communication defines three domains that were originally named production, explanation and aesthetics.[3] Doctors are most at home in the productive domain, where diagnoses and plans of action are made. They also constantly operate, knowingly or otherwise, in the domain of explanation or, as I would prefer to call it, that of interpretation. You might expect a doctor to keep the domain of aesthetics at arm's length, but it encompasses judgements of value that are crucial to illness experience. These include knowing illness as a bad feeling (see p. 36), as a state that is abnormal and therefore 'wrong' (see pp. 27 and 82). The dynamics of stigma is another aesthetic issue. The moral dimension of badness/wrongness, touched on in Chapters 5 and 6, also belongs in the domain of aesthetics. Conversely, a person's vision of well-being has an aesthetic aspect, and not a purely cognitive character.

Judgements of value are at the core of illness experience; they can only be recognized when a doctor moves from the domain of production to the domain of interpretation, but Anatole Broyard seems also to be calling for something more.

The ideal doctor, he says, 'would "read" my poetry, my literature. He would see that my sickness has purified me, weakening my worst parts and strengthening the best'; he wishes that his doctor 'would brood on my situation for perhaps five minutes, that he would give me his whole mind just once, be bonded with me for a brief space, survey my soul as well as my flesh, to get at my illness, for each man is ill in his own way'.[4] Siri Hustvedt is seeing her symptoms in an aesthetic light when she notices that 'tracking my pathology turns out to be an adventure in the history of experience and perception'.

How should we read a symptom or an illness?'[5] A doctor's reading is done within the domains of production, interpretation and also aesthetics, in order to achieve an empathic understanding of what is – in any or all of these senses – wrong. The outcome will be Broyard's 'poem of diagnosis'. However, a person cannot get much help towards positive possibilities until the doctor, the patient and others are able to obtain a shared vision of what is right.

Notes

1　The image of an offer comes from Balint 2000.
2　Kirmayer 2000
3　Lang et al. 1990
4　'The Patient Examines the Doctor' in Broyard 1992
5　Hustvedt 2011, p. 69

APPENDIX 1

TABLE 13.1 Index of Characters

Name	Age	Associated people	Chapter	Difficulties
Adèle	13	Bronwen (mother)	7	Mysterious, fluctuating symptoms
Adrian	52		9	Bladder problems (MS)
Alan	55		7	Severe impairments (MND)
Ali	17		6	Eating disorder
Bert	80		9	Rigid leg, acute illness + PD
Cheryl	75		8	Progressive neurological disability
Clio	17		8	Suicidal depression
Clive	44		6	Inability to stand (MS)
Daphne	40		6	Feeling guilty (MS)
Denis	58		7	Loss of independence (MS)
Diane	49		7	Impairments, social stresses (MS)
Dick	48		9	Unstable cyclist (HD)
Elaine	57		5	Unexplained loss of vision
Ethan	50		9	Potassium deficiency, paralysis
Eva	42		7	Severe impairments (MND)
Evan	14		5	Strange behaviour in the clinic
Faqar	42		7	Unable to express needs (HD)
Françoise	18		10	Recovering from brain injury
Gill	55		9	Multiple complex problems (MS)
Gordon	45		5	Unexplained loss of vision
Gwen	58		6	Symptoms suggest CFS/ME
Gwyneth	77		9	Stroke, severe walking difficulty
Henry	39		6	Once trapped in a burning building
Hugh	47		10	Disabling chronic pain
James	42	Margaret (wife)	8	Social isolation (HD)
Joe	29		10	Non-specific pains and lassitude
John	26		5	Non-epileptic seizures

(Continued)

Table 13.1 (Cont.)

Name	Age	Associated people	Chapter	Difficulties
Jordan	15	Shelley, George (parents)	6	Anxious, obsessive and erratic
Lena	72	Tomasz (husband)	8	Looked after in bed (MS)
Lori	35		5	Mysterious painful illness
Lucy	60		10	Suicidal depression
Madeleine	37		7	Motivated but frustrated by fatigue
Matteo	51	Sophia (daughter)	10	Severe impairments (MND)
Meg	51		9	Paraplegia, muscle spasms (MS)
Melanie	33	Dan (partner)	8	Physical impairments (MS)
Millie	89		8	Multiple symptoms
Moira	68		6	Mother of a woman with HD
Pat	63	Don (husband)	7	Progressive impairments (PD)
Paul	39		8	Multiple minor symptoms (MS)
Petra	60		9	Acutely ill (MND)
Rowena	4		5	Sudden onset of limping
Sam	30		5	Unable to walk, variable disability
Sarah	72		7	Stroke, physical problems, distress
Sinaid	34	Jock (partner)	10	Impact of diagnosis (MS)
Stuart	24		9	Head pains, 'wobbles'
Susie	70		5	Walking difficulty, variable
Violet	14		8	Disruptive behaviour (ASD)
Wahid	33		5	Paraplegia cured by hypnosis
Willie	35		5	Ostensibly diabetes and epilepsy
Yvonne	60		7	Severe impairments (MND)
Zola	31	Anna, her friend	Passim	Unspecified unwellness

Abbreviations for medical diagnoses: ASD = autism spectrum disorder; CFS/ME = Chronic fatigue syndrome or ME; HD = Huntington's disease; MND = motor neurone disease; MS = multiple sclerosis; PD = Parkinson's disease

BIBLIOGRAPHY

Abbott, A (1988). *The System of Professions: An Essay on the Division of Expert Labor*. Chicago: University of Chicago Press

Acheson, RA (1978). The definition and identification of need for healthcare. *Journal of Epidemiology & Community Health*, 32: 10–15

Adams, HE et al. (2002). The classification of abnormal behavior: an overview. In: PB SutkerHE Adams. *Comprehensive Handbook of Psychopathology*. 3rd Edn. New York: Kluwer Academic Publishers. Chapter 1

Adetunji, B et al. (2006). Detection and management of malingering in a clinical setting. *Primary Psychiatry*, 13: 61–69

Aggarwal, R et al. (2015). Distinctions between diagnostic and classification criteria. *Arthritis Care and Research (Hoboken)*, 67: 891–897

Ahmed, AA (2000). Health and disease: an Islamic framework. In: A Sheikh & AR Gatrad (Eds). *Caring for Muslim Patients*. Abingdon: Radcliffe Medical Press, Chapter 3

Aldwin, C & Igarashi, H (2012). An ecological model of resilience in late life. In: B Hayslip & GC Smith. *Annual Review of Gerontology and Geriatrics. Volume 32: Emerging Perspectives on Resilience in Adulthood and Later Life*. Chapter 6

Allen-Collinson, J & Pavey, A (2014). Touching moments: phenomenological sociology and the haptic dimension in the lived experience of motor neurone disease. *Sociology of Health & Illness*, 36: 793–806

Alonzo, AA (1985). An analytic typology of disclaimers, excuses and justifications surrounding illness: a situational approach to health and illness. *Social Science & Medicine*, 21: 153–162

APA (American Psychiatric Association) (2013). *Diagnostic and Statistical Manual of Mental Disorders (DSM–5)*. www.psychiatry.org/psychiatrists/practice/dsm

Anders, E (2014). Locating convalescence in Victorian England. *Remedia*, November 2014. https://remedianetwork.net/2014/11/07/locating-convalescence-in-victorian-england

Anderson, A & Goolishian, HA (1988). Human systems as linguistic systems: preliminary and evolving ideas about the implications for clinical theory. *Family Process*, 27: 371–393

Anderson, H et al. (1986). Problem determined systems: towards transformation in family therapy. *Journal of Strategic & Systemic Therapies*, 5: 1–13

Arikha, N (2007). *Passions and Tempers: A History of the Humours*. New York: Harper Perennial

Aristotle (2000). *Nichomachean Ethics*. R Crisp (Ed). Cambridge: Cambridge University Press

Asher, R (1951). Munchausen's syndrome. *Lancet*, 1: 339–341

Asher, R (1972). *Richard Asher Talking Sense*. London: Pitman Medical

Ashy, MA (1999). Health and illness from an Islamic perspective. *Journal of Religion and Health*, 38: 241–257

Atkinson, P (1997). *The Clinical Experience. The Construction and Reconstruction of Medical Reality*. 2nd Edn. Aldershot: Ashgate

Australian Institute of Health and Welfare (2018). Life expectancy and potentially avoidable deaths in 2014–2016. https://myhealthycommunities.gov.au/our-reports/life-expectancy-and-pad/july-2018

Ayo, J & Ayo, K (2008). *Body Matters: A Phenomenology of Sickness, Disease, and Illness*. Lanham: Lexington Books

Bachelard, G (1994). *Poetics of Space*. Transl. M Jolas. Boston: Beacon Press

Baker, G (2001). Wittgenstein: Concepts or Conceptions? *Harvard Review of Philosophy*, 9: 7–23

Bakhtin, MM (1986). *Speech Genres and Other Late Essays*. Transl. VW McGee, Eds C Emerson, M Holquist. Austin: University of Texas Press

Balint, J (2000). *The Doctor, His Patient and The Illness*. Ed 2. London: Churchill Livingstone/Elsevier

Barraclough, K (2004). Diagnosis and Wittgenstein's theories of language. *British Journal of General Practice*, 54: 480–481.

Bartholomew, RE (1994). Disease, disorder, or deception? Latah as habit in a Malay extended family. *The Journal of Nervous and Mental Disease*, 182: 331–338

Bartlett, FC (1932). *A Study in Experimental and Social Psychology*. Cambridge: Cambridge University Press

Bass, C & Halligan, P (2014). Factitious disorders and malingering: challenges for clinical assessment and management. *Lancet*, 383: 1422–1432

Bateson, G (2002). *Mind and Nature: A Necessary Unity*. Cresskill: Hampton Press

Becker, E (1973). *The Denial of Death*. New York: The Free Press

Beerbohm, M (1923). A home-coming. In: *Yet Again*. London: Heineman, Chapter 18

Bell, AM (2009). Approaching the genomics of risk-taking behavior. *Advances in Genetics*, 68: 83–104

Bennett, A (1995). *The Madness of King George*. Screenplay. New York: Random House

Bernanos, G (1937). *Journal of a Country Priest*. Transl. P Morris. London: Boriswood

Berryman, J (1969). *Dreamsongs*. New York: Farrar Straus and Giroux

Berryman, J (1973). *Recovery*. New York: Farrar, Straus and Giroux

Boszormenyi-Nagy, I & Krasner, BR (1986). *Between Give and Take. A Clinical Guide to Contextual Therapy*. New York: Brunner/Mazel

Boulding, KE (1956). General systems theory – the skeleton of science. *Management Science*, 2: 197–208

Bourdieu, P (1990). *The Logic of Practice*. Transl. R Nice. Cambridge: Polity Press

Bouveresse, J (1995). *Wittgenstein Reads Freud. The Myth of the Unconscious*. Transl. C Cosman. Princeton: Princeton University Press

Brown, CA (1841/1937). *The Life of John Keats*. Eds DH Bodurtha & WB Pope. London: Oxford University Press

Broyard, A (1992). *Intoxicated by My Illness: And Other Writings on Life and Death*. New York: Fawcett Columbine

Buddharakkhita, A (Transl.) (1996). The Dhammapada. The Buddha's Path of Wisdom. https://bit.ly/2RHKhX2

Burgler, E (1945). On the Disease-entity boredom ('alysosis') and its psychopathology. *Psychiatric Quarterly*, 19: 38–51

Burke, P (2012). *A Social History of Knowledge*. Cambridge: Polity Press

Bury, M (1982). Chronic illness as biographical disruption. *Sociology of Health and Illness*, 4:167–182

Canguilhem, G (1991). *The Normal and the Pathological*. Transl. CR Fawcett. New York: Zone Books

Cantor, C & Fallon, B (1996). *Phantom Illness: Shattering the Myth of Hypochondria*. Boston: Houghton Mifflin Harcourt

Carel, H (2013). *Illness. The Cry of the Flesh*. Revised Edition. Durham: Acumen

Cartwright, S (1851). Diseases and peculiarities of the Negro race. In: *De Bow's Review of the Southern and Western States*. Volume 11. New Orleans

Cerulli, A & Brahmadathan, UMT (2009). Know thy body, know thyself: decoding knowledge of the Aātman in Sanskrit medical literature. *eJournal of Indian Medicine*, 2: 101–107

Choquet, H & Meyre, D (2011). Genetics of obesity: what have we learned? *Current Genomics*, 12: 169–179

Clarke, JN & James, (2003). The radicalized self: the impact on the self of the contested nature of the diagnosis of chronic fatigue syndrome. *Social Science & Medicine*, 57: 1387–1395

Conrad, P (2007). *The Medicalization of Society: On the Transformation of Human Conditions into Treatable Disorders*. Baltimore: Johns Hopkins University Press

Coolidge, FL et al. (2007). Understanding madmen: a DSM-IV assessment of Adolf Hitler. *Individual Differences Research*, 5: 30–43

Corrigan, PW et al. (2009). Self-stigma and the 'why try' effect: impact on life goals and evidence-based practices. *World Psychiatry*, 8: 75–81

Coryllos, PN (1933). How do rest and collapse treatment cure pulmonary tuberculosis? *JAMA*, 100: 480–482.

Cromby, J (2015). *Feeling Bodies: Embodying Psychology*. London: Palgrave Macmillan

Cromby, J (2015b). The public meaning of CFS/ME: making up people. In: CD Ward (Ed). *Meanings of ME. Interpersonal and Social Dimensions of Chronic Fatigue*. London: Macmillan Palgrave. Chapter 9

Curth, LH (2003). Lessons from the past: preventive medicine in early modern England. *Medical Humanities*, 29: 16–21

Cutter, W (2011). *Midrash and Medicine. Healing Body and Soul in the Jewish Interpretive Tradition*. Woodstock: Jewish Lights

Daudet, A (2002). *In the Land of Pain*. Transl. J Barnes. London: Jonathan Cape

De Waal, F (2001). *The Ape and the Sushi Master: Cultural Reflections by a Primatologist*. New York: Basic Books

Deegan, P (1996). Recovery as a journey of the heart. *Psychiatric Rehabilitation Journal*, 19: 91–97

Department of Health, NHS England (2015). *Future in Mind*. NHS England https://bit.ly/2Kr7RTn

Derksen, F et al. (2013). Effectiveness of empathy in general practice: a systematic review. *British Journal of General Practice*, 63.76–84

Descartes, R (1637/1968). *Discourse on Method and other Writings*. Transl. FE Sutcliffe. London: Penguin Books

Diamond, JC (1998). *Because Cowards Get Cancer Too*. London: Vermilion

Dickson Wright, A (1955/1956). 'How patients have deceived me'. Presidential Address. *Transactions of the Hunterian Society*, 14: 13–30

Dinos, S et al. (2009). A systematic review of chronic fatigue, its syndromes and ethnicity: prevalence, severity, co-morbidity and coping. *International Journal of Epidemiology*, 38: 1554–1570

Douglas, M (1966/1984). *Purity and Danger. An Analysis of the Concepts of Pollution and Taboo.* London: Routledge

Duggan, JM & Duggan, AF (2006). *The Epidemiology of Alimentary Diseases.* Dordrecht: Springer

Duggleby, W et al. (2012). Hope, older adults, and chronic illness: a metasynthesis of qualitative research. *Journal of Advanced Nursing,* 68: 1211–1223

Dumit, J (2006). 'Illnesses you have to fight to get': facts as forces in uncertain, emergent illnesses. *Social Science & Medicine,* 62: 577–590

Dunlap, R (2016) Hope without the future: Zen Buddhist hope in Do-gen's Shobogenzo. *Journal of Japanese Philosophy* 4: 107–135

Edens, JF & Guy, LS (2001). Factors differentiating successful versus unsuccessful malingerers. *Journal of Personality Assessment,* 77: 333–338

Ehrenreich, B (2009). *Smile or Die: How Positive Thinking Fooled America & the World.* London: Granta

Elder, H (2015). Te Waka Oranga: bringing indigenous knowledge forward. In: K McPherson et al. (Eds). *Rethinking Rehabilitation. Theory and Practice.* Boca Raton: CRC Press, Chapter 12

Engel, G (1977). The need for a new medical model: a challenge for biomedical science. *Science,* 196:126–129

Epictetus (2nd century CE/1956). *The Discourses as Reported by Arrian. The Manual, and Fragments.* Transl. WA Oldfather. Loeb Classical Library. Cambridge: Harvard University Press

Epstein, M (2006). *Open to Desire. The Truth about What the Buddha Taught.* New York: Gotham Books

Farkas, M (2007). The vision of recovery today: what it is and what it means for services. *World Psychiatry,* 6: 68–74

Ferenczi, S (1926). The phenomena of hysterical materialization. Thoughts on the conception of hysterical conversion and symbolism. In: J Rickman (Ed). *Further Contributions to the Theory and Technique of Psycho-analysis.* Transl. JA Suttoe et al. London: Hogarth Press, 89–104

Field, BI & Reed, K (2016). The rise and fall of the mental health recovery model. *International Journal of Psychosocial Rehabilitation,* 20: 86–95

Fishman, A (2002). *Judaism and Collective Life. Self and Community in the Religious Kibbutz.* London: Routledge

Fonagy, P (2000). Attachment and borderline personality disorder. *Journal of the American Psychoanalytic Association,* 48: 1129–1146

Foucault, M (1978). *History of Sexuality. Volume 1: An Introduction.* Transl. R Hurley. New York: Vintage Books

Foucault, M (1988). Technologies of the self. In: LH Martin et al. (Eds). *Technologies of the Self. A Seminar with Michel Foucault.* London: Tavistock Publications, Chapter 2.

Fox, D et al. (Eds) (2009). *Critical Psychology: An Introduction.* London: Sage

Francis, G (2018). *Shapeshifters: On Medicine and Human Change.* London: Wellcome Collection, Profile Books

Frank, A (1997). *The Wounded Storyteller: Body, Illness and Ethics.* Chicago: University of Chicago Press

Frankl, V (1964). *Man's Search for Meaning. An Introduction to Logotherapy.* Transl. I Lasch. London: Hodder & Stoughton

Fredman, G (1997). *Death Talk. Conversations with Children and Families.* London: Karnac Books

Freud, S (1901/2002). *The Psychopathology of Everyday Life.* London: Penguin Books

Freud, S (1914–1916). *Some character-types met with in psycho-analytic work. The Standard Edition of the Complete Psychological Works of Sigmund Freud. Volume XIV.* London: Hogarth Press and the Institute of Psycho-Analysis

Freud, S (1919/2003). *The Uncanny*. Transl. D Mclintock. London: Penguin Books

Fukuda, K et al. (1994). International Chronic Fatigue Syndrome Study Group. The Chronic fatigue syndrome: a comprehensive approach to its definition and study. *Annals of Internal Medicine*, 121: 953–959

Furman, B (2010). *Kids' Skills in Action*. Victoria: Innovative Resources

Fürst, EL (2015). Coming back to oneself: a case of anoxic brain damage from a phenomenological Perspective. *Culture, Medicine and Psychiatry*, 39: 121–133

Furst, LR (2002). *Idioms of Distress. Psychosomatic Disorders in Medical and Imaginative Literature*. New York: SUNY Press

Geertz, C (1983). *Local Knowledge*. London: Fontana Press

Gilman, CP (1892). *The Yellow Wallpaper and Selected Writings*. London: Virago, 2009

Goffman, E (1956). *Presentation of Self in Everyday Life*. London: Penguin Books, 1990

Goffman, E (1968). *Stigma: Notes on the Management of Spoiled Identity*. New Jersey: Prentice-Hall

Good, BJ (2007). *Medicine, Rationality and Experience: An Anthropological Perspective*. Cambridge: Cambridge University Press

Griffith, JL (2010). *Religion that Heals, Religion that Harms: A Guide for Clinical Practice*. New York: The Guilford Press

Griffith, JL & Ryan, N (2015). Stigma, unspeakable dilemmas, and somatic symptoms - a legacy of in CFS/ME/ME and fibromyalgia. In: CD Ward (Ed). *Meanings of ME. Interpersonal and Social Dimensions of Chronic Fatigue*. London: Macmillan Palgrave, Chapter 12

Griffith, JL & Griffith, M (1994). *The Body Speaks. Therapeutic Dialogues for Mind-body Problems*. New York: Basic Books

Groves, JE (1978). Taking care of the hateful patient. *Lancet*, 298: 883–887

Guillermo, B (1980). Couple interactions: a study of the punctuation process. *International Journal of Family Therapy*, 2: 47–56

Hadot, P (1995). *Philosophy as a Way of Life. Spiritual Exercises from Socrates to Foucault*. Ed AI Davidson, Transl. M Vhase. Oxford: Blackwell, 1995

Harré, R et al. (2009). Recent advances in positioning theory. *Theory & Psychology*, 19: 5–31

Harvey, A et al. (2012). The future of technologies for personalized medicine. *New Biotechnology*, 29: 625–633

Harvey, K & Koteyko, N (2013). *Exploring Health Communication. Language in Action*. London: Routledge

Havi, C (2018). Invisible suffering: the experience of breathlessness. In: L Škof & P Berndtson (Eds) *Atmospheres of breathing: the respiratory questions of philosophy*. New York: SUNY Press, Chapter 15

Hawkes, N (2011). Dangers of research into chronic fatigue syndrome. *British Medical Journal*, 342: d3780

Heidegger, M (1962). *Being and Time*. Transl. J Macquarrie & E Robinson. Oxford: Blackwell

Hilton, J (1863/1950). *Hilton's Rest and Pain*. Eds EW Walls et al. London: G. Bell & Sons

Hinton, DE & Lewis-Fernández, R (Eds) (2010). Trauma and Idioms of Distress. Special Issue: *Culture, Medicine, and Psychiatry*, 34. 209–218

Hojat, M et al. (2009). The devil is in the third year: a longitudinal study of erosion of empathy in medical school. *Academic Medicine*, 84: 1182–1191

Holaday, B et al. (1994). Vygotsky's zone of proximal development: implications for nurse assistance of children's learning. *Issues in Comprehensive Pediatric Nursing*, 17: 15–27

Holgate, ST et al. (2011). Chronic fatigue syndrome: understanding a complex illness. *Nature Reviews (Neuroscience)*, 12: 539–544

Hollway, W (1984). Gender difference and the production of subjectivity. In: J Henriques et al. (Eds). *Changing the Subject: Psychology, Social Regulation and Subjectivity*. London: Methuen

Holmes, B (2010). *The Symptom and the Subject. The Emergence of the Physical Body in Ancient Greece*. Princeton: Princeton University Press

Horvarth, AO & Luborsky, L (1993). The role of therapeutic alliance in psychotherapy. *Journal of Consulting and Clinical Psychiatry*, 61: 561–573

Hurwitz, B & Bates, V (2016). The roots and ramifications of narrative in modern medicine. In: Whitehead, A, Woods A et al. (Eds). *The Edinburgh Companion to the Critical Medical Humanities*. Edinburgh: Edinburgh University Press, Chapter 32

Hustvedt, S (2011). *The Shaking Woman or A History of My Nerves*. London: Sceptre

ICAO (International Civil Aviation Organization) (2012). FRMS. Fatigue risk management system. Manual for regulators. ICAO https://bit.ly/2FFnlm9

Illich, I (1976). *Limits to Medicine. Medical Nemesis: The Expropriation of Health*. London: Marion Boyars

James, W (1890/1918). *Principles of Psychology in Two Volumes, Volume 1*. New York: Dover Publications

James, W (1905). *Varieties of Religious Experience. A study in Human Nature (Gifford Lectures 1901–1902)*. London: Longmans, Green & Co

Jason, LA et al. (2005). Chronic fatigue syndrome: the need for subtypes. *Neuropsychology Review*, 15: 29–58

Jelliffe, SE (1925). Somatic pathology and psychopathology at the encephalitis crossroads : a fragment. *Journal of Nervous and Mental Disorders*, 61: 561–586

Jewson, N (1976). The disappearance of the sick-man from medical cosmology 1770–1870. *Sociology*, 10: 225–244

Johnstone, L (2006). Controversies and debates about formulation. In: L Johnstone & R Dallos (Eds). *Formulation in Psychology and Psychotherapy*. London and New York: Routledge, Chapter 9

Joseph, CL (2018). Toward a black African theological anthropology and ubuntu ethics. *Journal of Religion and Theology*, 2: 16–30

Jureidini, J & Taylor, DC (2002). Hysteria. Pretending to be sick and its consequences. *European Child & Adolescent Psychiatry*, 11: 123–128

Khakpour, P (2018). *Sick. A memoir*. Edinburgh: Canongate

Kathol, RG (1997). Reassurance therapy: what to say to symptomatic patients with benign or non-existent medical disease. *International Journal of Psychiatry and Medicine*, 27: 173–180

Kelley, JM et al. (2014). The Influence of the patient-clinician relationship on healthcare outcomes: a systematic review and meta-analysis of randomized controlled trials. *PLoS One*. 9: e94207.

Kennedy, F (1926). The neuroses in the course of chronic epidemic encephalitis. *Archives of Neurology and Psychiatry*, 15: 515.

Kirkland, JL et al. (2016). Resilience in aging mice. *Journal of Gerontology – Series A*, 71: 1407–1414

Kirmayer, LJ (2000). Broken narratives: clinical encounters and the poetics of illness experience. In: C Mattingly & L Garro (Eds). *Narrative and the Cultural Construction of Illness and Healing*. Berkeley: University of California Press, 153–180

Klein, M (1952). Notes on some schizoid mechanisms. In: J Riviere (Ed). *Developments in Psychoanalysis*. London: Karnac, Chapter 9.

Kleinman, A (1988). *The Illness Narratives. Suffering, Healing, and the Human Condition*. New York: Basic Books

Koerner, J (2011). *Healing Presence: The Essence of Nursing*. New York: Springer Publishing

Korzybski, A (1994). *Science and Sanity. An Introduction to Non-Aristotelian Systems and Semantics*. Brooklyn: Institute of General Semantics

Krahé, C et al. (2015). Attachment style moderates partner presence effects on pain: a laser-evoked potentials study. *Scan*, 10: 1030–1037

Krause-Utz, A Elzinga, B (2018).   Current understanding of the neural mechanisms of dissociation in borderline personality disorder. *Current Behavioral Neuroscience Reports*, 5: 113–123

Laing, RD (1960). *The Divided Self.* London: Pelican Books

Laing, RD (1967). *The Politics of Experience & The Bird of Paradise.* London: Penguin Books

Laing, RD & Esterson, A (1970). *Sanity, Madness and the Family: Families of Schizophrenics.* London: Pelican Books

Lambert, MJ & Barley, DE (2001). Research summary on the therapeutic relationship and psychotherapy outcome. *Psychotherapy*, 38: 357–361

Lamma, C & Majdand, J (2015). The role of shared neural activations, mirror neurons, and morality in empathy – a critical comment. *Neuroscience Research*, 90: 15–24

Lang, WP et al. (1990). The systemic professional. Domains of action and the question of neutrality. *Journal of Systemic Consultation & Management*, 1: 39–55

Lask, B (2004). Pervasive refusal syndrome. *Advances in Psychiatric Treatment*, 10: 153–159

Lemert, C (2005). *Social Things. An Introduction to the Sociological Life.* 3rd Edn. Lanham: Rowman and Littlefield

Leplège, AC et al. (2015). Conceptualizing disability to inform rehabilitation: historical and epistemological perspectives. In: K McPherson et al. (Eds). *Rethinking Rehabilitation. Theory and Practice.* Boca Raton: CRC Press

Lewis, A (1975). The survival of hysteria. *Psychiatric Medicine*, 5: 9–12

Lewis, G (2010). *A Hospital Odyssey.* Newcastle: Bloodaxe Books

Lodge, D (1995). *Therapy.* London: Penguin Books

Loncraine, R (2018). *Skybound. A Journey of Flight.* London: Picador

Lorde, A (1980). *The Cancer Journals. Special Edition.* San Francisco: Aunt Lute Books

Lubbock, T (2012). *Until Further Notice I Am Alive.* London: Granta

MacEachen, E (2005). The demise of repetitive strain injury in sceptical governing rationalities of workplace managers. *Sociology of Health & Illness*, 27: 490–515

Malla, A et al. (2015). 'Mental illness is like any other medical illness': a critical examination of the statement and its impact on patient care and society. *Journal of Psychiatry & Neuroscience*, 40: 147–150

Mann, T (1922). *Buddenbrooks.* Transl. HT Lowe-Porter. London: Secker & Warburg. Part 9, Chapter 1

Mann, T (1928). *The Magic Mountain* [Der Zauberberg]. Transl. HT Lowe-Porter. London: Secker & Warburg

Mansfield, K (2006). *Journal of Katherine Mansfield.* London: Persephone Books

Mars-Jones, A & White, E (1987). *The Darker Proof: Stories from a Crisis.* London: Faber & Faber

Martin, K (2016). Modernism and the medicalization of sunlight: D. H. Lawrence, Katherine Mansfield, and the sun cure. *Modernism/Modernity*, 23: 423–441

Masolo, DA (2010). *Self and Community in a Changing World.* Bloomington: Indiana University Press

Maslow, AH (1987). *Motivation and Personality.* 3rd Edn. New York: Longman

Masten, AS (2001). Ordinary magic. Resilience processes in development. *American Psychologist*, 56: 227–238

Mauss, MA (1902/1972). *General Theory of Magic.* Transl. R. Brain. London: Routledge

Mayou, R (2014). Is the DSM-5 chapter on somatic symptom disorder any better than DSM-IV somatoform disorder? *British Journal of Psychiatry*, 204: 418–419

McHugh, PR & Slavney, PR (1986). *The Perspectives of Psychiatry.* Baltimore and London: The Johns Hopkins Press

Macnaughton, J & Carel, H (2016). Breathing and breathlessness in clinic and culture: using critical medical humanities to bridge an epistemic gap. In: A Whitehead & A Woods et al.

(Eds). *The Edinburgh Companion to the Critical Medical Humanities*. Edinburgh: Edinburgh University Press, Chapter 16

McPherson, S & Armstrong, D (2006). Social determinants of diagnostic labels in depression. *Social Science & Medicine*, 62: 50–58

McPherson, K et al. (Eds) (2015). *Rethinking Rehabilitation. Theory and Practice*. Boca Raton: CRC Press

Mechanic, D (1961). The concept of illness behavior. *Journal of Chronic Disease*, 15: 189–194

Mehmedinović, S (2012). My Heart. *Granta*, Issue 120

Meier, EA et al. (2016). Defining a good death (successful dying): literature review and a call for research and public dialogue. *American Journal of Geriatric Psychiatry*, 24: 261–271

Mercer, SW et al. (2016). General practitioners' empathy and health outcomes: a prospective observational study of consultations in areas of high and low deprivation. *Annals of Family Medicine*, 14: 117–124

Merleau-Ponty, M (2002). *Phenomenology of Perception*. Transl. C Smith. London: Routledge

Merrell, F (2001). Charles Sanders Peirce's concept of the sign. In: P Cobley (Ed). *The Routledge Companion to Semiotics and Linguistics*. London and New York: Routledge, Chapter 2

Merton, R (1976). *Sociological Ambivalence and Other Essays*. New York: The Free Press

Miller, J (1978). *The Body in Question*. London: Jonathan Cape

Mills, CW (1959/2000). *The Sociological Imagination*. Oxford: Oxford University Press

Mitchell, SW (1899). *Fat and Blood*. Philadelphia: JB Lippincott Company

Mitchell, W (2017). *Someone I Used to Know*. London: Bloomsbury

Modell, H et al. (2015). A physiologist's view of homeostasis. *Advances in Physiology Education*, 39: 259–266

Moerman, DE. (2002). *Meaning, Medicine and the 'Placebo Effect'*. Cambridge: Cambridge University Press

Mohr, DC et al. (2004). Association between stressful life events and exacerbation in multiple sclerosis: a meta-analysis. *British Medical Journal*, 328: 731

Muscio, B (1921). Is a fatigue test possible? *British Journal of Psychology*, 12: 31–36

Natelson, BH (2008). *Your Symptoms are Real: What to Do When the Doctor Says Nothing is Wrong. Overcoming Pain, Fibromyalgia, Chronic Fatigue, IBS, and More*. Hoboken: John Wiley & Sons

Newson, E et al. (2003). Pathological demand avoidance syndrome: a necessary distinction within the pervasive developmental disorders. *Archives of Disease in Childhood*, 88: 595–600

Newton, H (2017). 'She sleeps well and eats an egg': convalescent care in early modern England. In: S Cavallo & S Storey (Eds). *Conserving Health in Early Modern Culture: Bodies and Environments in Italy and England*. Manchester: Manchester University Press, Chapter 4

NHS Digital (2016). *Mental Health and Wellbeing in England: Adult Psychiatric Morbidity Survey 2014*. https://bit.ly/2LoqXNf

NICE (National Institute for Health and Clinical Excellence) (2007). *Clinical Guideline 53 – Chronic fatigue syndrome/myalgic encephalomyelitis (or encephalopathy): diagnosis and management of CFS/ME in adults and children*. www.nice.org.uk/guidance/cg53

NICE (2013). Dementia: independence and wellbeing. www.nice.org.uk/guidance/QS30

Nightingale, DJ & Cromby, J (2001). Critical psychology and the ideology of individualism. *Journal of Critical Psychiatry and Psychotherapy*, 1: 117–128

Nijdam-Jones, A (2017). A cross-cultural analysis of the test of memory malingering among Latin American Spanish-speaking adults. *Law and Human Behavior*, 41: 422–428

Occhi, D (1999). Sounds of the heart and mind: mimetics of emotional states in Japanese. In G Palmer & DJ Occhi (Eds), *Languages of Sentiment: Cultural Constructions of Emotional Substrates*. Amsterdam: John Benjamins Publishing Company, 151–170

Oliver, D (2008). 'Acopia' and 'social admission' are not diagnoses: why older people deserve better. *Journal of the Royal Society of Medicine*, 101: 168–174.

Oliver, M (1996). *Understanding Disability. From Theory to Practice*. New York: Macmillan Education

Orwell, G (1946/2006). *Politics and the English Language*. Peterborough: Broadview Press

Parsons, T (1964). *The Social System. The major exposition of the author's conceptual scheme for the analysis of the dynamics of the social system*. New York: The Free Press

Patterson, SW (2010). 'A picture held us captive': The later Wittgenstein on visual argumentation. *Cogency*, 2: 105–134

Pearce, JMS (2004). Silas Weir Mitchell and the 'rest cure'. *Journal of Neurology, Neurosurgery, and Psychiatry*, 75: 381.

Peirce, CS (1931–1966). *Collected Papers*. Eds C Hartshorne et al. Cambridge: Belknap

Peng, K & NisbettRE (1999). Culture, dialectics and reasoning about contradiction. *American Psychologist*, 54: 741–754

Pessoa, F (1991). *The Book of Disquiet*. Transl. MJ Costa. London: Serpent's Tail

Picardie, R (1998). *Before I Say Goodbye*. London: Penguin Books

Pickstone, JV (2000). *Ways of Knowing: A New History of Science, Technology and Medicine*. Manchester: Manchester University Press

Plantinga, C. (1995). *Not the Way it's Supposed to Be: A Breviary of Sin*. Grand Rapids: William B. Eerdmans Publishing

Polanyi, M (1958). *Personal Knowledge*. London: Routledge & Kegan Paul

Porter, KA (1939/1965). Pale horse, pale rider. In: *The Collected Stories of Katherine Anne Porter*. New York: Harcourt, Brace & World, Chapter 3

Porter, R (1997). *The Greatest Benefit to Mankind: A Medical History of Humanity*. New York and London: WW Norton

Power, RA & Pluess, M (2015). Heritability estimates of the Big Five personality traits based on common genetic variants. *Translational Psychiatry*, 5: e604

Proust, M (1920/1982). *Swann's Way. Volume 2: The Guermantes Way*. Transl. CK Scott Moncrieff & T Kilmartin. New York: Random House

Pullman, D (2002). Human dignity and the ethics and aesthetics of pain and suffering. *Theoretical Medicine and Bioethics*, 23: 75–94

Quain, R (1895). *A Dictionary of Medicine*. New York: D. Appleton and Company

Radley, A (1999). The aesthetics of illness: narrative, horror and the sublime. *Sociology of Health & Illness*, 21: 778–796

Ramaswamy, C (2016). *Expecting*. Salford: Saraband

Ramsay, DS & WoodsSC (2014). Clarifying the roles of homeostasis and allostasis in physiological regulation. *Psychological Review*, 121: 225–247

Rantzen, E (2000). No cause, no cure. *Nursing Standard*, 14: 23.

Riadore, JE (1843). *Treatise on Irritation of The Spinal Nerves as the Source of Nervousness, Indigestion etc and on the Modifying Influence of Temperament and Habits of Man over Diseases*. London: J Churchill

Rudebeck, CE (2000). The doctor, the patient and the body. *Scandinavan Journal of Primary Health Care*, 18: 4–8

Rumsey, N et al. (1982). The effect of facial disfigurement on the proxemic behavior of the general public. *Journal of Applied Social Psychology*, 12: 137–150

Ryan, RM & Deci, EL (2018). *Self-Determination Theory. Basic Psychological Needs in Motivation, Development, and Wellness*. New York: Guilford Press

Sacks, O (1986). *A Leg To Stand On*. London: Picador

Sacks, O (1992). Tourette's syndrome and creativity: exploiting the ticcy witticisms and witty ticcicisms. *British Medical Journal*, 305: 1515–1516

Sartre, J-P (1938). *La Nausée*. Paris: Gallimard

Saunders, L (2015). The challenge of CFS/ME in primary care. In: CD Ward (Ed). *Meanings of ME. Interpersonal and Social Dimensions of Chronic Fatigue*. London: Macmillan Palgrave, Chapter 10

Scarry, E (1985). *The Body in Pain: The Making and Unmaking of the World*. Oxford: Oxford University Press

Scott, S (2006). The medicalisation of shyness: from social misfit to social fitness. *Sociology of Health & Illness*, 28: 133–153

Sedgwick, P (1982). *Psycho Politics*. London: Pluto Press

Shakespeare, T (2018). *Disability. The Basics*. London: Routledge

Showalter, E (1997). *Hystories: Hysterical Epidemics and Modern Media*. New York: Columbia University Press

Siedentop, L (2015). *Inventing the Individual: The Origins of Western Liberalism*. London: Penguin Books

Slater, L (2000). *Lying*. London: Penguin Books

Smith, GC & Hayslip, B (2012). Resilience in adulthood and later life. What does it mean and where are we heading? In: B Hatalip & GC Smith (Eds). *Annual Review of Gerontology and Geriatrics. Volume 32: Emerging Perspectives on Resilience in Adulthood and Later Life*. Chapter 1

Smith, JEH (2017). *Embodiment. A History*. Oxford: Oxford University Press

Smith, WC (1998). *Believing – An Historical Perspective*. Oxford: Oneworld

Sontag, S (1978). *Illness as Metaphor*. New York: Farrar, Straus and Giroux

Stacey, M (1988). *The Sociology of Health and Healing*. London: Unwin Hyman

Standen, PJ et al. (2015). Symptoms into words: how medical patients talk about fatigue. In: CD Ward (Ed). *Meanings of ME. Interpersonal and Social Dimensions of Chronic Fatigue*. Basingstoke: Macmillan Palgrave, Chapter 6

Sulloway, F (1979). *Freud, Biologist of the Mind: Beyond the Psychoanalytic Legend*. Cambridge: Harvard University Press

Svenaeus, F (2011). Illness as unhomelike being-in-the-world: Heidegger and the phenomenology of medicine. *Medicine, Health Care and Philosophy*, 14: 333–334

Sydenham, T (1665/1848). Medical observations concerning the history and cure of acute diseases. In: *The Works of Thomas Sydenham*. Translated from the Latin Edition of Dr Greenhill by RG Latham. London: The Sydenham Society; C and J Adlard, Section 1, Chapter 1

Temkin, O (1963). The scientific approach to disease: specific entity and individual illness. In: AC Crombie (Ed). *Scientific Change: Historical Studies in the Intellectual, Social and Technical Conditions for Scientific Discovery and Technical Invention from Antiquity to the Present*. New York: Basic Books, 629–647

Thomas, KB (1987). General practice consultations: is there any point in being positive? *British Medical Journal*, 294: 1200–1202

Trnka, S (2007). Negotiating the 'real' and the relational in Indo-Fijian women's expressions of physical pain. *Medical Anthropology Quarterly*, 21: 388–408

Tutu, D (2011). *God is Not a Christian. Speaking Truth in Times of Crisis*. New York: HarperOne with London: Rider Books

Ulrich, RS (1984). View through a window may influence recovery from surgery. *Science*, 224: 420–421

Van der Kolk, B (2014). *The Body Keeps the Score: Brain, Mind, and Body in the Healing of Trauma*. London: Penguin Publishing Group

Vanstone, WH (1982). *The Stature of Waiting*. London: Darton, Longman and Todd

Von Bertalanffy, L (1972). The history and status of general systems theory. *Academy of Management Journal*, 15: 407–426

Von Uexküll, J (1934/2010). *A Foray Into the Worlds of Animals and Humans: With a Theory of Meaning*. Transl. JD Neil. Minneapolis/London: University of Minnesota Press.

Vuilleumier, P (2005). Hysterical conversion and brain function. *Progress in Brain Research*, 150: 309–329

Wakefield, J (2007). The concept of mental disorder: diagnostic implications of the harmful dysfunction analysis. *World Psychiatry*, 6: 149–156

Wall, D (2005). *Encounters with the Invisible. Unseen iIlness, Controversy, and Chronic Fatigue Syndrome*. Dallas: Southern Methodist University Press

Ward, CD (2008). Symptoms in society: the cultural significance of fatigue. In: A Morgan (Ed). *Being Human. Reflections on Mental Distress in Society*. Ross-on-Wye: PCCS Books, Chapter 9

Ward, CD (2012). Is patient-centred care a good thing? *Clinical Rehabilitation*, 26: 3–9

Ward, CD (Ed) (2015) *Meanings of ME. Interpersonal and Social Dimensions of Chronic Fatigue*. London: Palgrave Macmillan

Ward, CD (2015a). Ibid Chapter 3: Scientifically speaking: CFS/ME in the medical literature, 26–33

Ward, CD (2015b). Ibid Chapter 11: The said and the unsaid: ambivalence in CFS/ME, 165–176

Ward, CD (2015c). Ibid Chapter 13: What does the diagnosis say?, 198–212

Ward, CD (2015d). Ibid Chapter 14: Ways of Not Knowing, 213–225

Ward, CD et al. (2011). Using systemic approaches, methods and techniques in rehabilitation medicine . *Clinical Rehabilitation*, 25: 3–13

Ware, NC (1999). Toward a model of social course in chronic illness: the example of chronic fatigue syndrome. *Culture, Medicine and Psychiatry*, 23: 303–331

Warrell, DA et al. (Eds) (2010). *Oxford Textbook of Medicine*. Oxford: Oxford University Press.

Watzlawick, P et al. (1974). *Change. Principles of Problem Formation and Problem Resolution*. New York, London: WW Norton & Company

Weingarten, W (2010). Reasonable Hope: Construct, Clinical Applications, and Supports. *Family Process*, 49: 5–25

Weintrobe, S (2013). *Engaging with Climate Change: Psychoanalytic and Interdisciplinary Perspectives*. London: Routledge

Weiss, E (2011). Widening the boundaries. In: W Cutter (Ed). *Midrash and Medicine. Healing Body and Soul in the Jewish Interpretive Tradition*. Woodstock: Jewish Lights

Whitehead, L (2006). Quest, chaos and restitution: Living with chronic fatigue syndrome/ myalgic encephalomyelitis. *Social Science and Medicine*, 62: 2236–2245

WHO (World Health Organisation) (1948). Constitution. www.who.int/about/who-we-a re/constitution

WHO (1976). *International Classification of Impairments, Disabilities, and Handicaps. A Manual of Classification Relating to the Consequences of Disease*. http://apps.who.int/iris/bitstream/ 10665/41003/1/9241541261_eng.pdf

WHO (2001). *International Classification of Functioning, Disability and Health*. www.who.int/cla ssifications/icf/en

WHO (2013). *International Classification of Functioning, Disability and Health Draft Practical Manual*. www.who.int/classifications/drafticfpracticalmanual2.pdf?ua=1

WHO (2016) *International Classification of Diseases (ICD-10)*. https://icd.who.int/browse10/ 2016/en

Williams, AT et al. (2013). Novel genetic variants associated with lumbar disc degeneration in northern Europeans: a meta-analysis of 4600 subjects. *Annals of Rheumatic Diseases*, 72: 1141–1148

Williams, AC de C & Craig, KD (2016). Updating the definition of pain. *Pain*, 157: 2420–2423

Williams, AC de C & Johnson, M (2011). Persistent pain: not a medically unexplained symptom. *British Journal of General Practice*, 61: 638–639

Williams, S (2000). Chronic illness as biographical disruption, or biographical disruption as chronic illnes? Reflections on a core concept. *Sociology of Health & Illness*, 22: 40–67

Winnicott, C (2016). D.W.W.: a reflection. In: R Shepherd (Ed). *The Collected Works of D. W. Winnicott: Volume 12, Appendices and Bibliographies*. Oxford: Oxford University Press

Winnicott, DW (1990). *Home is Where We Start From: Essays by a Psychoanalyst*. London: Penguin Books

Winnicott, DW (2005). *Playing and Reality*. London: Routledge

Wittgenstein, L (1967). *Philosophical Investigations* [Philosophische Untersuchungen]. Transl. GEM Anscombe. Oxford: Basil Blackwell

Wittgenstein, L (1977). *On Certainty* [Über Gewissheit]. Transl. D Paul, GEM Anscombe. Oxford: Basil Blackwell

Wittgenstein, L (1980). *Culture and Value*. Transl. P Winch. Chicago: University of Chicago Press

Wolterstorff, N (1983). *Until Justice and Peace Embrace*. Grand Rapids: William B. Eerdmans Publishing

Wong, VW et al. (2013). Wound healing: a paradigm for regeneration. *Mayo Clinic Proceedings*, 88: 1022–1031

Woolf, V (1926). *On Being Ill*. https://thenewcriterion1926.files.wordpress.com/2014/12/woolf-on-being-ill.pdf

Zautra, AJ et al. (2010). Resilience: promoting well-being through recovery, sustainability, and growth. *Research in Human Development*, 7: 221–238

INDEX

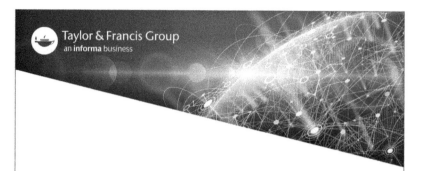

Milton Keynes UK
Ingram Content Group UK Ltd.
UKHW031151141024
449569UK00024B/877